Master Gao Yun • Master Bai Yin

Qigong Energy Healing
"Five Elements Rejuvenation Therapy"

The Personal Program to Heal and Strengthen Your Life Energy with
Sounds, Diet, Mudras, Timing, and the Five Rejuvenation Exercises

Translated by Christine M. Grimm

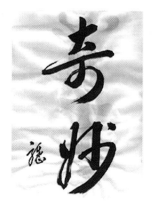

"The wonders of Qi"

LOTUS PRESS • SHANGRI-LA

The information introduced in this book has been carefully researched and passed on to the best of our knowledge and conscience. Despite this fact, neither the authors nor the publisher assume any type of liability for presumed or actual damages of any kind that might result from the direct or indirect application or use of the statements in this book. The information in this book is intended for interested readers and educational purposes. It is not intended to be understood as instructions for therapy or diagnosis in the medical sense. All serious health disorders and any symptoms that may have a serious illness as their cause should definitely be diagnosed and treated by a naturopath or medical professional.

First English Edition 2001
©by Lotus Press, Box 325
Twin Lakes, WI 53181, USA
The Shangri-La Series is published in cooperation
With Schneelöwe Verlagsberatung, Federal Republic of Germany
©2000 by Windpferd Verlagsgesellschaft mbH, Aitrang, Germany
All rights reserved
Translated by Christine M. Grimm
Cover design by Kuhn Graphik, Digitales Design, Zurich, Switzerland
Drawings by Daniel Muschalik (pg. 36-42, 44, 54)
Calligraphies by Ning Wang, page1: Bay Yin
Illustrations by Peter Krafft, Designagentur, Freiburg, Germany with drawings by Diana Krafft (pg. 28-29)

ISBN 0-914955-69-1

Printed in Germany

How You Can Benefit Most from This Book
in the Shortest Amount of Time

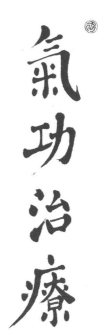

Two recognized Qigong masters will lead you into the fundamentals of qigong. Dr. Gao Yun is a well-known qigong master who has already introduced hundreds of thousands of people to qigong. Together with her daughter Master Bai Yin, she teaches and heals throughout the world.

The qigong exercises, methods of diagnosis, and life principles presented here are based on the five elements. The theory of the five elements runs throughout the entire book. Page by page, you will become increasingly more familiar with this system of classifying all of the life processes. The energy of the fire, earth, metal, water, and wood elements will pervade you—and you will experience them. In the process, you will gradually discover how you are a part of these forces with your physical strengths and weak points, as well as your mental vitality.

You will be actively initiated into the possibilities for stimulating your powers of self-healing, which will increasingly strengthen your own qi force. The ancient Chinese already knew that a disturbed flow of qi is the root of all illness. And so the qigong energy healing affects the qi from a great variety of directions in order to let it flow abundantly once again.

At the same time, qi codes are the key to finding the qi blocks. These qi codes can be used as a diagnostic instrument on the one hand; but they are also useful because they have the potential of transforming harmful qi into healing qi. You can learn to immediately put these possibilities to practical use in the chapter on "Healing with the Qi Code of the Five Elements" on pg. 15 ff. It will show you how to easily located your special problem area and then discover which energy exercises are especially suitable for you. As you do this, there is nothing that you can do wrong because the activated qi flows exactly to wherever it is needed.

The five healers of the qi code are: sound, music, optimal timing, nutrition, and a lifestyle in harmony with the five elements. The mudras and the Five Element Rejuvenation Exercises form the heart of this book. These particularly powerful exercises correspond with the five elements and the five "qi animals." These short exercises sequences are easy to learn, yet result in extensive positive effects. These can be further intensified when the exercises are practiced in the corresponding atmosphere of sound.

The energy and powers of self-healing that are released in this process are part of the field of energetic medicine—which many people already consider the healing art of the future.

We wish you much enjoyment in learning and practicing these exercises!

Table of Contents

CHAPTER 1

The Magic of Natural Healing

Five Natural Methods of Healing

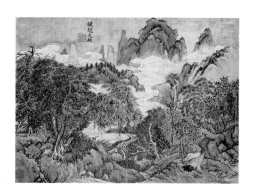

In our striving for physical, mental, and emotional health, can we human beings depend upon doctors to successfully treat all of our diseases? Conventional Western medicine uses isolated measures for controlling specific health disorders: for example, insulin is administered against diabetes, antibiotics prescribed against inflammation, and hysterectomies performed on women with fibroids in the uterine wall. This type of treatment often disregards the fact that the various prescribed medications can cause allergic or toxic reactions, which in turn lead to other complaints. Although the afflicted areas of the body are brought under control and/or completely removed, new problems continue to develop as a result.

We live in a polluted environment. The quality of our lives is continually deteriorating, causing us to become ill. In most cases, conventional Western medicine has not yet found a genuine solution for relieving pain and truly healing health disorders. Although the world of medical science has introduced new technologies for the treatment of disease, it simultaneously causes other diseases. Because of its effectiveness without the use of drugs and development of side effects, the naturopathic method of qigong healing has gained recognition throughout the world: It has given people new hope and renewal in their lives.

In our current age, people are increasingly seeking natural methods of healing. They are learning techniques for taking care of their own lives, increasing their inner vital energy and preventing their complaints from worsening in order to promote a sound mind and healthy body. For more than 30 years, we have been involved with this topic. More than 300,000 people have attended our courses during this time and we have supported them in applying the various natural methods of healing to improve their health. We believe that this alternative healing method will become *the* new trend of the 21st Century.

As life continues to evolve, human beings still follow the laws of the earth. In turn, the earth follows the laws of the universe: heaven and earth follow the laws of nature. The elements of nature therefore become the laws of nature that we should obey. We can therefore use these elements to precisely determine and correct physical disturbances.

The laws of the universe

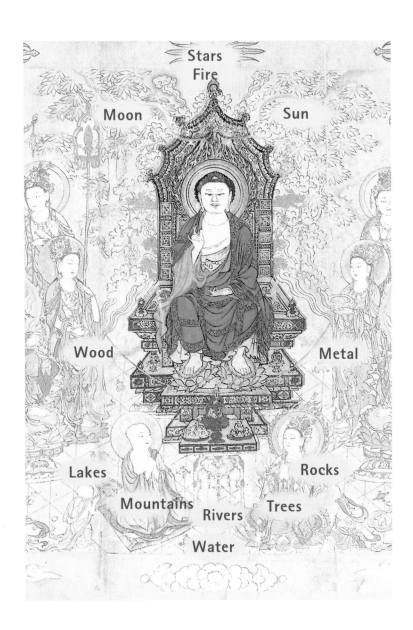

In our many years of research, we have discovered that mental healing, nutritional healing, energy healing, massage, healing with water, healing with movement, healing with music, and aromatherapy are the most effective natural methods of healing.

We believe that everyone can achieve outstanding health and an abundant supply of qi with the following five factors: healing of the mind, healing of the qi, magnetic healing, nutritional healing, and healing through medical treatment. These five factors correspond to the Chinese "five elements" and fulfill the basic requirements for complete and holistic health.

Healing of the five elements

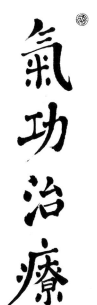

Healing of the mind:
Achieving happiness and inner peace
through continual correction
of our mental and emotional life
is the basis for maintaining health.

Healing through movement:
Proper daily exercise
is the key to keeping
our energy flowing
and helps clear away blocks.

Healing through nutrition:
Food contains natural substances
and nutrients.
Eating a proper and balanced diet
can improve the state of health.

Qi energy healing:
The lack of vital energy can be
compared with a tree that doesn't
have enough roots or water that doesn't flow.
Increasing the level of this energy
is the precondition for our health.

Medical treatment:
Regular check-ups
and timely treatment
contribute to maintaining
our physical health.

This book provides information on how to achieve optimal health by using the effective holistic methods of the qi and the five elements. These are methods that regulate the bodily processes from within and ultimately help us achieve the highest goal of self-healing.

Master Gao Yun

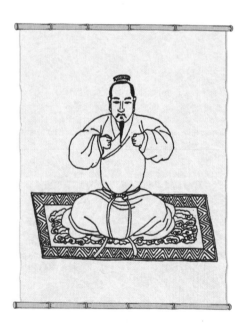

CHAPTER 2

The Qi Code of Energy Healing

The Fundamentals of Holistic Healing

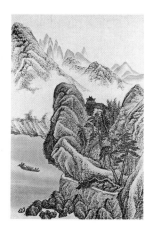

Qi—The Essence of the Life Force

According to the ancient Chinese perspective, qi is the basic force that is contained in all life forms and required to sustain life. In addition, it exists in the universe, in the heavens and on earth, as well as in all living creatures. Even though qi cannot be touched or detected by the naked eye, it still exists everywhere.

If we look at the entire universe, qi is contained in the vast mountains and scenic rivers, as well as in the world of plants and animals. The respective level of qi reflects the type of life force and strength of any object or being.

The same kind of qi also fills our bodies. It may be strong or weak—depending on how well we manage to supply and nourish it. This qi also rules over our life span and determines our personality, our passions and emotions. We believe that qi dominates our entire lives from birth to sickness and from aging to death.

The bioenergy "qi" is the primordial force for the development of life

Life begins at the moment of conception in the mother's womb, and the internal energy is also formed at that very moment. After birth, we absorb nutrients from our food and through the intake of water and oxygen. The internal qi is the combination of our inherited prenatal qi and the absorption of food, water, and air. These two elements form the absolutely essential internal bio-energy required for sustaining life. This internal bio-energy of "qi" is the basic force for the development of life, as well as the fundamental element of our body. In this respect, qi is also called the "primordial essence." If the body is adequately supplied with it, it becomes strengthened. Conversely, if the internal qi is weakened, disease will occur; when it is exhausted, the result is death.

Qigong—A Medical Alternative

We can study qigong as a method for using the qi to achieve healing in a variety of ways. In terms of its effectiveness, it offers the same benefits as conventional Western medicine; namely, healing health disorders and maintaining physical health. However, it is apparent that medical qigong is distinctly different from conventional medicine in both theory and practice. Conventional medicine treats our bodily diseases while medical qigong attempts to resolve the problems and afflictions associated with the body, mind, and soul. Western medicine mainly relies on injections, medications, and surgical procedures when treating illness. But it hasn't yet found a way of explaining or controlling the fate to which the body is subjected.

The primordial essence

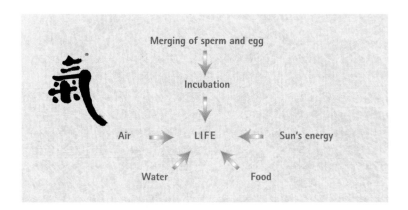

Qigong begins with the principle of strengthening the life force. The prevention of disease before it even develops by regulating the qi and improving blood circulation are the main forms of qigong treatment. The most effective methods for preventing and healing disease are a combination of medical qigong, conventional medicine, and a practice of continually strengthening the life energy.

These are Essential Components of the Daily Practice for Strengthening the Life Energy.

The main goal of qigong is to establish a better lifestyle in order to achieve a healthy body and alert mind. The first step toward this goal is attaining a good state of health, which then strengthens the body/mind. The practice of

How Do We Strengthen the Life Energy?

For the ancient Chinese, this was a familiar topic and virtually part of their everyday practice. Examples of this are:
• How and when to go to bed and get up
• How to eat and what we should wear
• How to prolong our life
• How to strengthen various parts of the body and help them adapt to demands placed on them
• How to achieve vibrant physical health
• How to maintain a youthful appearance
• How to attune ourselves to heaven and earth

qigong helps us attain good health by relieving emotional anxiety and mental agitation, transforming and sublimating it on a spiritual level.

Qigong has an effect on the body, soul, and mind

We can benefit from the practice of qigong since it allows us to heal ourselves without resorting to conventional medical treatment and surgical procedures. When our pain and suffering is relieved, we can appreciate life even more. This permits us to take a path of confidence in life. These naturopathic methods of healing are actually alternative medical approaches that we can depend on.

Diagnosis of Illness through Telepathic Perception of Qi

Long-time qigong practitioners often experience the free flow of qi within their body. Their internal organs are filled with positive and spiritual qi. At a certain level, their body will be permeated with qi. This can be seen in their visible aura, flowing from the crown of the head. This force is powerful enough to heal others upon contact—it is even capable of exorcising evil. We consider this to be the highest level of qigong.

When the human body becomes ill, there is a lack of qi. This deficiency is usually located in the painful or wounded area and the aura displays a pale, opaque color or a layer that looks like black smoke. The clearest examples of this can be seen in people who have just undergone surgery or patients with a brain tumor. Under normal circumstances, healthy people have a 2.5 inch thick layer of white qi that hovers around their head (1). On the other hand, the area where a brain tumor has been removed shows a dark indentation (3). This is another technique for determining the existence of health disorders through the telepathic perception of qi. The examples below give us an idea of how the qi energy and qi deficits can be perceived.

1
Health and abundant qi

2
Frequent illness with deficient qi

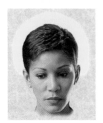 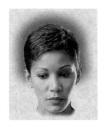 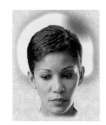

3
Brain tumor directly after operation

Disruption of Qi as the Trigger for Illness

Some people feel pain and discomfort without knowing what type of illness they have contracted. They frequently suffer from headaches, shoulder pain, backaches, and related problems with the spine. What causes all of these problems? They are actually caused by a disruption of the qi.

When a disorder of the qi occurs in the body, a variety of complaints can develop. The blocked channels of the qi cause obstructions to occur, and these obstructions cause pain.

In simple terms: An obstruction of qi is expressed as pain, which is caused by blockages

Nie Jing, the ancient Chinese book of medicine, states that: "All diseases are caused by the disorder of the qi." External factors for this are, for example, the flu and other epidemics; the internal factors are the diminished and/or exhausted qi. The disorder of the qi occurs at the place where the problem is located. Such disorders can be divided into three categories: deficiency of the qi, obstruction of the qi, and inversion of the qi.

• *Deficiency of the qi:*

Prolonged illness, premature aging, and extreme fatigue will lead to a deficiency of the qi. Examples of the related symptoms are general weakness and shortness of the breath, a flat and toneless voice, lack of appetite, digestive disorders, weak bladder, spermatorrhea, and an increased susceptibility to infectious diseases.

The qi becomes blocked within the body, which can be compared to a traffic standstill. When this occurs, the meridians (energy channels) in the body become blocked, all of the organ functions are disturbed and begin to stagnate. This state is usually indicated by the following symptoms: shoulder and back pain, a swollen abdomen because of excessive waste qi, sore feeling in the chest, and sagging of the lower abdomen.

• Obstruction of the qi:

The qi travels in the opposite direction. This condition is normally associated with the lungs and stomach. Symptoms include coughing, asthma, nausea, vomiting, and hypertension.

• Inversion of the qi:

The practice of qigong has the goal of strengthening our inner qi so that it is filled with power and vibrancy. When this powerful force flows through the pathways of the meridians, it has an igniting and energizing effect. It supplies the entire body with positive qi. If we can correct the three problem areas listed above, we can prevent and/or eliminate all complaints.

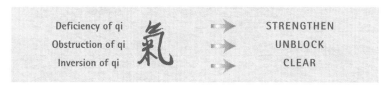

Correction of the qi imbalance

Deficiency of qi		STRENGTHEN
Obstruction of qi		UNBLOCK
Inversion of qi		CLEAR

Changing Harmful Qi into Healing Qi

The primary form of qigong practice is the technique of regulating and expanding our inner qi. This qi is commonly referred to as the "primordial essence" or "intrinsic vital energy" that exists and circulates within our entire body.

Traditional Chinese Medicine (TCM) believes that the occurrence of disease and pathological disorders can be explained through the theory of "healing and harmful qi."

Healing qi is the primordial essence, an element that regulates our physical body and supports the proper metabolism and functioning of the immune system. On the other hand, malignant or harmful qi corresponds with the toxic elements in our body, which initially cause functional disorders and eventually lead to diseases.

Healing or harmful qi determines whether the body is healthy or sick. When the healing qi prevails, it can normally prevent the occurrence of disease. This state can be seen in the healthy body. Otherwise, the opposite circumstance will develop.

Which method can we use to enrich this primordial essence? How can we free ourselves of the harmful qi? How can we maintain and restore the positive qi within our body? These are the profound questions related to the qi code of the five elements and the practice of qigong. They will be discussed within the scope of this book.

From the Nei Jing: "Securing the primordial qi can prevent negative factors from intruding into our bodily system."

Healing qi

Adapting to nature	**HEALING QI**	Metabolism
Preventing disease		Physiological harmonization

Harmful qi

Functional disorders	**HARMFUL QI**	Sickness
Early death		Mental disease

CHAPTER 3

Healing with the Qi Code of the Five Elements

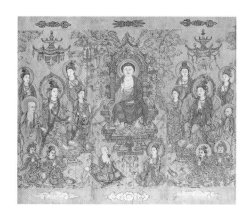

The Theory of the Five Elements

The ancient Chinese believed that the universe is made of five elements, each with unique characteristics. These are: wood, fire, earth, metal, and water, which are formed in this order.

The theory of the five elements refers not only to the existence of the elements of wood, fire, earth, metal, and water; they are also separated into five main categories according to their respective natures. The theory of the five elements is based on understanding how all manifestations of the universe can be integrated into these five categories. Typical characteristics indicate that everything belongs to a specific element, as illustrated in the following examples:

- **Fire** has a hot and rising character.
- **Earth** has an ability to plant, grow, and transform.
- **Metal** has a downward and renewing character.
- **Water** has a wet and cold character.
- **Wood** has a growing and ascending character.

According to the theory of Traditional Chinese Medicine (TCM), the fundamental study of human pathology and psychology, diagnosis, treatment, prescription of medication, and nutritional rules is closely related to the principle of the five elements. The human body corresponds with nature and is therefore part of the universal creation that follows the laws of cycles and transformation. The theory of the five elements also includes our inner vital organs, the tissue of the body, the five sensory organs, and the emotions.

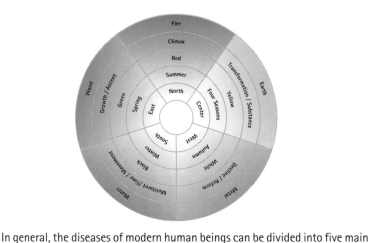

The characteristics of the five elements

The table below can help us to discover the cause of an illness or properly treat complaints that we already understand

In general, the diseases of modern human beings can be divided into five main groups according to the five elements. These are *the fire group, earth group, metal group, water group, and wood group*. In addition, according to TCM: "The organs hidden inside are reflected in the outer signs." This means that checking the respective surface organ can disclose the state of the afflicted internal organ. Through long years of research and scientific study, the ancient Chinese discovered that the five elements, the internal organs, the external organs such as the body parts (tongue, nose, mouth, ears, and eyes) and the structural organs or tissue (blood vessels, muscles, skin, bones, and tendons) are all interrelated. The internal organs provide the outer organs and the structural organs with nutrients. As a result, the weak or strong functional capacity of an internal organ is reflected in the respective external part of the body and in the tissue. In the form of symptoms or functional disorders, all of these signs will be exhibited in a very specific external or structural organ.

Element	Fire	Earth	Metal
Internal Organ	Heart, Small Intestine	Spleen, Stomach	Lungs, Large Intestine
External Organ	Face	Lips	Body Hair
Sensory Organ	Tongue	Mouth	Nose
Structure	Blood Vessels	Muscles	Skin
Emotion	Pleasure, Joy	Anxiety, Brooding	Sadness, Grief

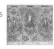

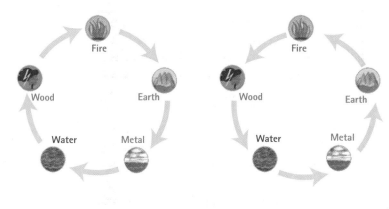

1. Generation: Beneficial influence on growth, development, and prolongment (clockwise)

2. Subjugation: Regulating influence on excessive or disorderly development (counterclockwise)

All manifestations in the universe are interrelated with the main five elements. Through connection with the five elements in the form of a network, they mutually influence and control each other. These elements create a system of order within the body and are related to each other in the manner of generation and subjugation. This relationship between generation and subjugation is also applied in TCM.

The two diagrams above show the following: One element influences the next element in the specific order of a mother-son relationship. This means that if the previous (or "mother") organ is ill, this will be passed on to the following (or "son") organ. In the reverse direction, when the son organ is weakened it can also influence the mother organ. Within the five-element system, each element has a specific relationship with the other four elements. Any two elements respectively will react to each other with some form of generation or subjugation in order to achieve proper control and balance in this manner. Consequently, when one of the organs becomes ill, this will cause harm to the entire system and throw it out of balance.

Element	Water	Wood
Internal Organ	Kidney, Bladder	Liver, Gallbladder
External Organ	Hair	Fingernails
Sense	Ears	Eyes
Structure	Bone	Tendons
Emotion	Fear	Anger

The five elements and their corresponding organs

17

How You Can Determine Your Element Group

The best way to make practical use of this book is to first find your problem area and symptoms in the following summary (pages 19 and 20). Then you will be able to place yourself in the correct element category. This is very easy to do: first, determine with which group a weakened area of the body is associated. This weakened organ will correspond with the element that you are lacking and which needs to be strengthened immediately.

How to get the greatest benefit from this book

If, for example, you notice that your symptoms are associated with those in the fire category, it means that your life force has a deficiency—or excess— of the "fire" element. This indicates your element or group

Then you may choose to use the appropriate qi code of natural healing methods for your element group, which will be introduced in the following chapter. In the process, you may also naturally discover that your symptoms are related to more than one group. This isn't unusual because the human body is a holistic system. One weakened organ reflects the functions of another organ and can create equilibrium between the organs. In such a case, you should refer to subsequent chapters such as "Diagnosing Illness through Interpretation of Physical Signs" or "Diagnosing Illness with Sound" to determine and confirm your element group.

How to Discover Your Weak Areas

Follow the five-step program:
1. First compare the columns of the following summary with each other to determine the element group for your symptoms or weak areas.
2. If you determine that your weak areas belong to more than just one element group, turn to the chapter on "Diagnosing Illness through Interpretation of Physical Signs", page 23-24 in order to precisely determine your element group.
3. Please be sure to only classify yourself in one element group that is most closely related to the majority of your symptoms or best describes your basic characteristics. This is your primary or main element.
4. Five unique methods of natural healing are presented in this book. They are: healing with sound, healing with timing, healing with the qi code of nutrition, healing with the hands and fingers through certain types of mudras, and—the most effective technique—healing with five-element qigong for rejuvenation.

5. You may first begin any of the above healing techniques with your primary and main element. Then follow the path of generation for the five elements (see page 17, above). Then practice the next element, and so forth.

Element	Symptoms or Weak Areas
Fire Group 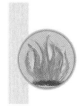	Insomnia, hypertension, poor memory, hypothyroidism, shoulder or back pain, chest pain, heart disease, arrhythmic palpitation, neurasthenia, dizziness, shortness of breath, weakness, lack of myocardial oxygen, excessive phlegm, soreness of arms, nightmares, dry mouth, stiff tongue.
Earth Group 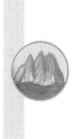	Excessive flatulence, gastritis, stomach ulcer, gastroptosis, duodenal ulcer, anorexia, ascites, vomiting, stomach ache, fatigue, poor digestion, functional disorders of stomach and spleen, constipation, chronic hepatitis, stroke, diabetes, cancer, rheumatoid arthritis, cancer of the colon, gallstones, eating disorders that may include excessive hunger; deficient intake of food leads to inadequate qi and blood.
Metal Group 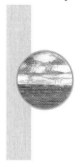	Susceptibility to flu, poor immune response, heavy breathing during movement, dull and hoarse voice, sore and swollen throat, inability to hold prolonged conversations, low and deep vocal chords in women, high and weak vocal chords in men, bronchitis, bronchial enlargement, nasal allergy, stuffy nose, excessive phlegm, gasping, frequent sneezing, runny nose, dry skin and dry hair, excessive wrinkling, frequent development of hemorrhoids, respiratory problems.

Summary for determining your element group

Water Group

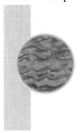

Disorders of sexual functions in men and women, impotence, premature ejaculation, irregular menstruation, frigidity, inability to conceive, nephritis, lower back pain, chilly feeling in abdomen, weak bladder, polyuria, cystitis, deterioration of hearing, tinnitus, both legs weakened, sore and aching body, loosening of bones and aching bones.

Wood Group

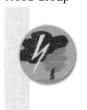

Bad moods, worry and depression, restlessness, deterioration of vision, premature presbyopia, teary eyes, dry eyes; iris that is grainy, itchy, or red; improper functioning of the liver due to excessive medication, enlargement of the liver, gallstones; back pain, stiff back and shoulders, fatigue.

Diagnosing Illness through Interpretation of Physical Signs

According to the holistic principle in Traditional Chinese Medicine (TCM), our internal organs and viscera should not be seen as isolated; in fact, they are closely connected with each other. The functions of each individual organ are reflected in the external state of the body. Examples of this are the color of the face, appearance, vitality, breath, and body odor

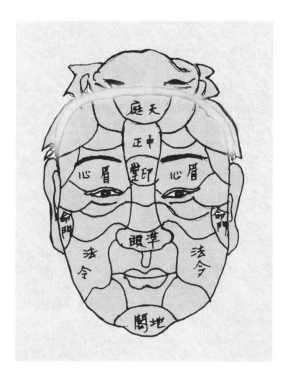

Instructions for diagnosing illness from the face

The techniques for diagnosing health problems by means of visual contact are the main emphasis of TCM. In earlier times, people believed that the highly developed master/doctor could discover impending disease before it occurred. As discussed in the previous chapter, when a vital organ becomes ill or disturbed in its function, this will be revealed at an external location on the body. The diagnosis of disease through visual contact is used to determine whether there are abnormalities in a person's physical condition. This includes the color and texture of the skin, the luster of the face and tongue, as well as posture and physical agility.

For example, a stuffy and pale-looking nose indicates problems in the respiratory system. Problems with the spleen or stomach are most likely expressed through bad breath and opaque lips. If the whites of the eyes become yellowish, this represents a problem that has developed in the liver and may possibly be related to jaundice, etc.

By adopting this method, an experienced doctor can precisely pinpoint the type and nature of the problem. TCM doctors use various diagnostic techniques such as visual contact, smell, feel, questions, and taking the pulse. I would also include the technique of qi diagnosis: in this approach, telepathic perception is used to determine the ailing area of the patient through the qi leaving the body in the form of the aura, its color, and intensity.

In its science of human beings, Chinese philosophy came to the conclusion that there are also five categories of people according to the body shape, luster and color of the face, etc. These are fire, earth, metal, water, and wood. Ancient Greek medicine showed that there are four fluid substances within the human body and divided them into four types of people: sanguine, melancholic, choleric, and phlegmatic. Modern psychology has divided human beings into five different basic types on the basis of the various secretions in our endocrine system: the thyroid type, the parathyroid type, the adrenal type, the pituitary type, and the sexual type. Some important characteristics of the different types of people in the ancient Chinese theory of the five elements are listed below.

Diagnosis using the properties of external body signs is also done on the basis of the five-element classification

When we connect the medical theory and the practice of interpreting the body signs with each other, we can determine the character and the personality, as well as the state of health, for any human being. Since all people are divided into five categories, the first step is to recognize your own type of character and the associated element. Every individual can be classified with one of the five elements on the following chart. Once you have determined what type you are, you can learn how to use your own qi to regulate your body, mind, and soul, your internal organs and viscera, as well as your diet and daily activities.

Diagnosing illness through interpretation of the body signs

Fire Type

Body form	– thin
Face shape	– angular, sharp
Face color	– red flushed
Voice	– rough
Sensory organs	– compact
Personality	– restless

Earth Type

Body form	– fat, big belly
Face shape	– large, round
Face color	– yellowish
Voice	– low, deep
Sensory organs	– strong, well-proportioned
Personality	– persevering

Metal Type

Body form	– muscular, firm belly
Face shape	– square, even
Face color	– clear, white
Voice	– high
Sensory organs	– even
Personality	– honest, faithful

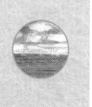

Water Type

Body form	– narrow shoulders, fat or thin
Face shape	– supple, round
Face color	– pale or white
Voice	– soft, mild
Sensory organs	– round, full
Personality	– easy-going

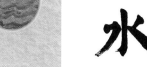

Wood Type

Body form	– long, thin
Face shape	– longish, narrow
Face color	– brownish
Voice	– clipped, clear
Sensory organs	– elongated
Personality	– kind

Comparative Overview: The Five-Element Typology

Fire	*Earth*	*Metal*	*Water*	*Wood*

Facial and Physical Attributes

Fire	Earth	Metal	Water	Wood
Small, red face, wide shoulders	Yellowish face, large and round, big belly, excessive fat, short height	Small head and flat belly, whitish face, high forehead, big bones	Opaque-appearing face, many wrinkles, large head, narrow shoulders, large abdomen, tall and thin	Longish facial form, light-brown color, sturdy shoulders, long and rigid body

Characteristics

Fire	Earth	Metal	Water	Wood
Passionate, easily excited, impatient, short-tempered, brave, intelligent, pioneering, ambitious, arrogant, very extroverted, favors cold, dislikes hot	Gentle, stable, peaceful, patient, tenacious, consistent, slow pace in thinking and acting, introverted	Generous and magnanimous, far-sighted, agile, talent for organization, calm, hypo-critical, adequate self-esteem, fanfare	Thoughtful, strategic mind, cunning, insincere, sly, depressive, extremely introverted	Talented, diligent, active, nimble, competent, good at public relations, extroverted, unstable, sensitive, suspicious

Susceptibility to Disease

Fire	Earth	Metal	Water	Wood
Cardiovascular problems, normal life expectancy	Spleen, problems with digestive system, long life expectancy	Problems with the lungs and respiratory system, average life expectancy	Kidney problems, long life expectancy	Liver problems, medium body strength, average life expectancy

Diagnosing Illness through Sound

As we have seen in the previous sections of this chapter, even though each of us has a different appearance, we can still be classified within one of the five element types. We should therefore attune and harmonize our body, mind, and soul to the type of element to which we belong. The following sections of this chapter describe how to integrate nutrition, music, work, exercise, and other practical aspects into our daily activities.

Follow the path to harmony

When the sound of the voice changes, this is an external sign that represents the internal organ—just like a change in the sound of a machine indicates that a problem is developing. Changes in the sound of the voice, in the form of coughing or moaning, are among the important warning signs of an impending disease.

Examples of this are the change to a higher or lower pitch, a more long-winded or shorter, slower or quicker way of speaking. These are alarm signals coming from the organs and viscera. In general, a firm and sonorous voice indicates healthy organs; an unclear and timid voice represents weak organs; a garbled sound reflects a disturbance of the sexual functions, as well as a lack of bodily qi. Diseases of the spleen normally are expressed in a slow voice, kidney diseases are reflected in a deep voice, lung disease is heard in a hasty voice, heart complaints in a high-pitched voice, and liver disease in a halting voice.

The pitch of the voice and its changes are signs of possible physical complaints

For many years now, we have used music as a remedy to channel the qi for healing purposes. We were astounded to learn that the treatments with music are extremely beneficial and their results very positive. We have therefore included the TCM theory of interaction between the five sounds and the five organs in our work. By tuning the five sounds to the five organs, harmonious music will enhance and stimulate the chemical reactions within the body by creating positive effects for curing disease. The feedback of the signals in our psychological and physiological context of mind/body is constantly adjusted and compared because any positive or negative input from outside elements will have an influence on the changes within the body.

Sound of Voice	Location of Disease in Respective Organ
• Long-winded, garbled	• Liver, gallbladder
• High pitch	• Heart, blood veins
• Slow, heavy	• Stomach, spleen
• Loud, fast	• Lungs, respiratory system
• Low, deep	• Kidneys, bladder

Diagnosing illness through sound

Healing with the Qi Code of Music

Since the sound of the voice reflects the—strong or weak—state of the internal organs, the proper function of these organs can be influenced by the use of the right music. The influx of sound and the frequencies of the internal organs connect with each other and resonate together. This gradually regulates the physiological body and attunes it to the proper, harmonious synchronization. Consequently, music is a spiritual force. During mental training, our body dances to the rhythm of the music and opens up our passions, an act comparable to birds flying into the sky.

Music generally has the effect of uplifting the emotions. Pleasant music leads to a positive and tranquil state of mind. It cleanses and purifies the spirit and improves the functioning of the vital organs. Conversely, loud and disharmonious sounds can cause adverse effects to the mind and the emotions. Pleasant, harmonious music therefore supports the flow of qi. Different types of sounds and melodies can affect our minds and emotions, change the rhythm of the breath, the heartbeat, and the brain waves. Music can be used to relieve conditions of fatigue. The music of the European middle ages and Eastern Buddhist music are similar in a certain sense: They both have a healing power and a positive influence on the way we live our lives.

Suitable music for every type of element

Music with the power to heal can be divided into five categories: You can choose the music that belongs to your type of element in order to fine-tune your body.

Music Fills the Room with Healing Power

For years we have held lectures and conducted seminars on natural healing throughout the world. We have taught each exercise together with the specific use of music. Prior to the start of the class, the room's atmosphere is filled with the healing power of music. This imparts pleasant signals to the central nervous systems of the students. Music can invigorate the inner qi. In this case, music becomes a dominant factor that leads to spiritual power during the group practice session. It becomes an especially important component when the characteristics of the five elements of music and the theory of medicine are combined to create new techniques for diagnosing and healing diseases.

Music can strengthen the inner qi and trigger healing reactions

In 1997, a qigong performance at the Frankfurt Book Fair touched the hearts of the audience with its graceful movements and beautiful music. This led to the good fortune of producing a special series of qigong music. Produced by the well-known musician and composer Andreas Mock especially for this purpose, this music series is called *Elements of Rejuvenation*. It conveys a healing effect to both the listener and the practitioner of qigong. This special album of music is designed to send positive signals to each vital organ. Each of the five-element rejuvenation exercises enables the qi to penetrate more deeply into our organs and cleanse the viscera in our organism. It also regulates the related organ functions when we use the body positions, colors, sound, timing, and shapes formed by the mouth and hands for the purpose of healing. As you listen to each piece of music with a relaxed body and total concentration, visualize the images that the music brings to mind and follow the melody of the song. This will enable you to completely connect with the artistic concept and ultimately experience an enhancement of your life.

Fire Music for the Circulatory System

The rhythm of fire music is joyful, lively, vital, and relaxing. It has a fiery power to it. It helps clear blocks and congestion in the veins and arteries, relieves tightness in the chest, shortness of breath, coughing, and excessive phlegm. Fire music also promotes the metabolism and improves the circulatory system.

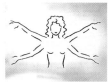

Example:

Composition No. 6 from

Elements of Rejuvenation—Transformation (Fire)

This composition, used together with the Flamingo Exercise (which will be introduced in a later chapter), is meant to strengthen the body's immune defense. Since the brain plays a leading role in this process, positive signals are sent to the brain when the mind focuses on the sensory stimulation of the melody. The result is beneficial stimulation of the brain. Together with the Flamingo Exercise, this piece of music especially emphasizes the act of rising and spreading our wings in a gentle and graceful manner. Imagine flying up into the sky, free of all bonds.

Earth Music for the Digestive System

The Earth Music has a gentle, festive, and elegant character with a floating sensation. Its strength and firmness is like the nature of the earth. Earth Music is especially intended for treating injury or weakness of the spleen and stomach. It supports the stimulation of the digestive system, improvement of the appetite, an increase and toning of the circulation for qi and blood.

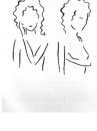

Example:

Composition No. 7 from

Elements of Rejuvenation—Devotion (Earth)

This special composition emphasizes the swiftness and agility of a little monkey. When doing the Monkey exercise (which will be introduced in a later chapter), imitate the characteristics of a monkey to achieve the best healing results.

Metal Music for the Respiratory System

This music is usually associated with high tones; it sounds impressive, serious, and solemn. It is intended for those who are afflicted with respiratory problems, a lack of mental concentration, and a chronic sense of coldness in the body.

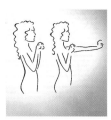

Example:

Composition No. 8 from

Elements of Rejuvenation—Cheerfulness (Metal)

This composition facilitates the absorption of the natural energy that we need for all bodily functions. It helps accelerate the elimination of negative energy through the metabolism and regulate the qi within the body, as well as cleansing it.

Water Music for the Urinary and Reproductive System

The melodies of the Water Music are very distinct, heavy, soft, and amiable. It is designed to relieve problems associated with the kidneys, enhance the hearing, and increase mental acuteness. In addition, it helps against tinnitus, insomnia, irritation, excessive dreaming, and hypertension.

Example:
Composition No. 9 from
Elements of Rejuvenation—Mysteriousness (Water)
This composition is designed especially for the Bear Exercise. It helps regulate and strengthen the kidneys and bladder. TCM believes that the growth, development, and reproduction of life are connected with the essences in the kidneys. This exercise concentrates on sexual dysfunctions and impediments, impotence, premature ejaculation, soreness in the legs and back, diabetes, and related health disorders.

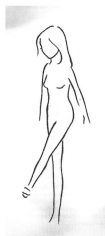

Wood Music for the Blood-Vessel System

This music with its sentimental, soft, and refreshing sounds has a healing power for problems related to the liver, for people who frequently suffer from stress, restlessness, and nightmares. It also helps prevent senile disorders.

Example:
Composition No. 10 from *Elements of Rejuvenation—Gentle Impulse (Wood)*
This composition is designed to accompany the Deer Exercise. It serves to regulate the liver and gallbladder. TCM believes that the liver fulfills the main function in the metabolic process. This exercise therefore focuses on the qi and blood, bringing relief to our emotions so that we can maintain a peaceful state of mind.

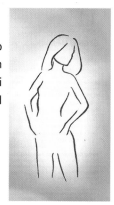

Healing with the Qi Code of Timing

Human beings are constantly affected by the changes in the universe. Consequently, each of us should abide by the laws of nature in order to survive. There is a simple analogy for this: When the temperature drops, we dress warmly. When it gets dark outside, we go to bed. When the sun rises, we get up again. When we violate the laws of nature, problems develop and our health deteriorates. The systems of the human body are linked to the laws and timing of nature. In this regard, one of the most important rules is related to the time plan of meridian circulation.

Things happen according to time and the laws of nature

Each day has 24 hours. When we divide this number by 2, we have 12 segments for each day. Since there are 12 meridian lines in the human body, these 12 time segments affect their proper circulation. According to ancient Chinese philosophy, "things happen according to time and the laws of nature." If we properly adapt to the laws of nature and the alternating circulation in yin-yang, we can live a healthier life with a longer life expectancy. The human body responds to heaven and earth. This also applies to our qi and our blood, which is subject to the time segments and changes in our environment. For example, the lung meridian is most active between 3 and 5 a.m.; between 7 and 9 a.m., the stomach meridian is most productive. As a result, asthma seizures usually occur in the early morning hours, heart attacks normally occur around noon, and other pain or afflictions also occur at a specific time of day or night. In summary, we could say that the conditions of the body are closely related to the order of the time segments and the laws of nature.

Exercise effectiveness is increased at certain times of the day

For people who frequently exercise, the fundamental physical condition is an indication for choosing the correct time segment. Exercising during that particular time segment will optimally intensify the effectiveness of the exercise. If we follow the principles related to the proper time segment, we will enjoy the benefits of harmonizing the body with the laws of nature. The following practical advice has been compiled according to the theory of "circulation of yin and yang in the body" under the aspect that observing the right time of day serves to prolong life.

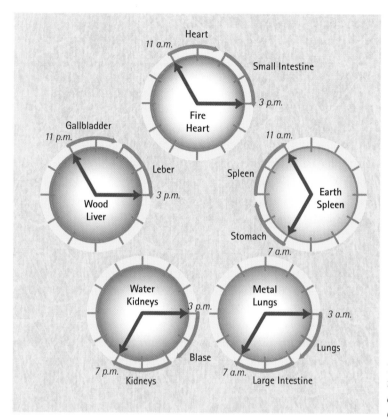

Time segments of the five elements and their related organs

• *Fire People—With Weak Nerves and Heart Conditions:*

Avoid eating too quickly and excessively at lunch. This will prevent heart complaints from developing. People with a weak heart will experience dizziness and drowsiness if they eat too much at lunchtime. We therefore suggest that you do not eat a full meal at that time and be sure to rest for about 30 minutes after the meal to improve the heart's condition. This group of people should avoid exercise or the practice of qigong between 11 a.m. and 1 p.m.

• *Earth People—With Digestive Problems:*

The most active time of the day for the stomach and spleen is between 7 a.m. and 11 a.m. This means that the metabolic activity of the stomach and the spleen, upon which the body depends, achieves peak efficiency during this time period. These people are advised to eat a good, nutritious breakfast since skipping breakfast is a bad habit and may eventually contribute to poor health. For this group of people, the ideal time segment for exercising is 5 a.m. to 7 a.m.

• *Metal People—With Respiratory Problems:*

It is advisable to get up early and perform deep breathing exercises in the fresh air. The respiratory system functions most actively between 5 a.m. and 7 a.m. Practicing qigong during this time segment counteracts constipation problems and is helpful as a preventive measure against lung cancer.

• *Water People—With Problems of the Urinary/Reproductive System*

The exercises should be performed between 3 p.m. and 7 p.m. This is the best time of day to replenish the qi in the body, which then improves and strengthens the kidney functions. People who suffer from lower back pain, frequent urination, and a reduced sexual ability should avoid sexual activities during this time segment to prevent further harm to the kidneys.

You can find the best time for qigong exercises here

• *Wood People—With Poor Blood Formation and Circulation*

Do not go to sleep any later than 11 p.m. since the respective problems will otherwise be intensified. The sleep between 11 p.m. and 3 a.m. is ideal for improving the system functions.

If you are afflicted by two or more problems from the above areas, the best time for exercise or qigong practice is either between 5 a.m. and 7 a.m. or between 7 p.m. and 9 p.m.

Healing with the Qi Code of Nutrition

Modern people tend to eat and drink much more than they need to. Poor dietary habits can ultimately harm our health. Two important aspects should be considered when eating: to eat correctly and to have the proper portions of the food.

Even the Chinese emperor in the 4th century had a nutritional advisor

The Chinese pay a great deal of attention to the nutritious value of food and the art of food preparation. They have derived certain principles of cooking through many years of experience. Already in the 4th Century, Chinese emperors appointed so-called "food consultants" to design special recipes with a balanced diet for the nobility. They believed that absorbing the proper first-rate nutrients from the food was essential for the growth and proper functioning of the body: This approach was intended to preserve the best possible state of health. Conversely, improper nutrition can become a source of health disorders.

The affluence of modern society and the convenience of fast foods, which contributes to a hectic and stressed lifestyle, leads people to choose the wrong types of foods. Most diseases are caused by the wrong food choices and unsanitary foods. "The mouth is the source of viruses" is a Chinese proverb. According to TCM's theory of the five elements, a well-prepared diet contributes more healing power for certain ailments.

The Relationship Between Taste and Organs

The ancient Chinese food consultants emphasized the interaction between the five tastes and the five organs. Foods are generally divided into five categories: s*weet, sour, bitter, salty, and spicy*. The intake of the five tastes into our organism has a direct influence on the internal organs. This effect can be beneficial or harmful, depending upon the amount and type of food intake.

For example, the sweet taste is connected with the spleen and stomach; the spicy taste is connected with the lungs and large intestine; the sour taste is connected with the liver and gallbladder; the bitter taste is connected with the heart and small intestine; and the salty taste is connected with the kidneys and bladder. When we understand the principles of the five tastes and the five organs, we can nourish the five organs in the right way. If any one of the five tastes is consumed excessively, it will damage the related organ. For example, too much of the sweet taste harms the stomach and spleen. This in turn leads to problems like a stuffy feeling in the head and chest, a sour taste in the mouth, coughing, and ulcers.

Light meals increase life expectancy

Through the years, we have studied and mastered a series of techniques that connect proper diet with qigong energy healing. This method can be used to treat problems in the energy channels and the qi/blood circulation. It also strengthens the functional systems of the tendons and bones, as well as the vital organs. The preventive qi within the body is enhanced as a result, and the nutrient qi is replenished. Both types of qi, preventive and nutrient qi, are essential substances for supplying the five vital organs and six viscera. They also promote longevity.

Our philosophy is that it is better to eat a diet that is light and simple instead of an abundance of heavy foods. Statistics show that people with a light intake of food over a certain period of time generally have a longer life expectancy than those who do not follow this principle.

Healing effect by eliminating certain foods from the diet

We prefer a diet of foods that contain phyto-nutrients, which possess healing properties. In general, these are vegetables, fruit, beans, and soy products, supplemented by fresh fish, seafood, and meat. Many vegetables contain protein, carbohydrates, sugar, and the vitamins necessary for good health. In addition, they provide micro-constituents that may contribute to controlling obesity and circulatory diseases by dilating prematurely constricted blood vessels. When we eat 500 or more grams of vegetables every day, this truly benefits our health.

However, we do not advise you to restrict the types of food you eat. Abstaining from certain types of foods is a practice for patients in a phase of acute illness and during the period of recuperation. During such times, patients should pay particular attention to their diet and abstain from foods that they should avoid. This approach is intended to prevent the disease from becoming protracted and/or worsened. .

How and when should we abstain from certain types of foods? For example, patients with tuberculosis should avoid spicy foods so that the lungs are not additionally burdened. Edema patients should strictly control their intake of salt to prevent excessive strain on the kidneys. People with a weak liver should avoid alcohol, and those with stomach ailments should not eat frozen or deep-fried foods. Certain medications should not be taken together with tea or grapefruit juice since toxic reactions may otherwise occur.

The Best Food

The best food comes from nature, as TCM emphasizes. The human diet and nutrient intake should naturally come from the five basic forces of nature. We divide foods according to the five elements. For example, there are five types of grains, each of which will enrich the respective organ and attune it when absorbed by the body. We believe that the scientific approach to nutrition should combine natural sources of food with a balanced diet.

The Colors of Food Are Also Important

Vegetables are also divided according to the five colors: red, yellow, white, green, and black. When vegetables are eaten in the proper ratio of the five colors to each other, this can be considered a well-balanced diet that supports the correct attunement of the five vital organs. In the West, black vegetables such as eggplant, black mushrooms, algae, and seaweed are not part of the normal diet. On the other hand, Orientals prefer black-colored vegetables because they contain ingredients with a tonic effect on the kidney function.

The following diagram shows the detailed connection of each element with the vital organs and the types of vegetables. According to your element group, you can make the best choice. Please remember that this is only a suggestion for a balanced diet. You don't have to just eat the primary element foods, but you should give a stronger preference to them in your daily nutritional plan.

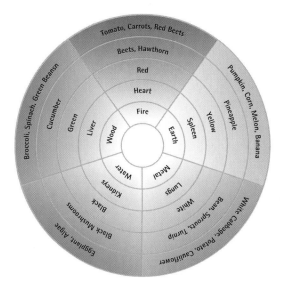

Healing food according to the theory of the five elements

Healing Foods for Fire People

Health Disorders or Chronic Complaints Related to the Element of "Fire"

Hypertension, cardiovascular disease, senile disorders, stroke, cerebral congestion, arrhythmia, irregular palpitation, chest pain, hyperthyroidism, Parkinson's disease, insomnia, poor memory, shoulder and back pain.

Foods with Healing Properties for "Fire":

- *Grain:* Rice, macaroni, wheat bread
- *Legume:* Chick peas
- *Vegetable:* Tomato, carrot, red beets, snow peas, potato, broccoli, green mustard, red peppers
- *Meat:* Deep-sea fish, shrimp, duck
- *Fruit:* Apple, pear, peach, plum, apricot, pineapple, orange, watermelon.
- *Foods to Avoid:* Meat with a high cholesterol content, animal internal organs, ham, salty fish, alcoholic beverages, coffee, carbonated soft drinks.

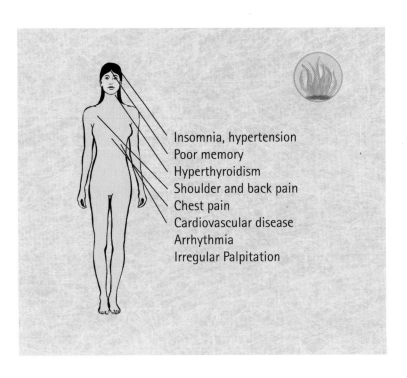

Insomnia, hypertension
Poor memory
Hyperthyroidism
Shoulder and back pain
Chest pain
Cardiovascular disease
Arrhythmia
Irregular Palpitation

Healing Foods for Earth People

Health Disorders or Chronic Complaints Related to the Element of "Earth"

Indigestion, stomach ache, poor appetite, bad breath, stomach ulcer, gastroptosis, stomach cancer, diabetes, muscle weakening.

Foods with Healing Properties for "Earth"

- *Grain:* Various and rich grain dishes for breakfast, wheat, oatmeal for easy digestion.
- *Vegetable:* Turnip, white cabbage, potato, pumpkin, ginger, carrot, corn, mushroom, onion, pepper, linseed, squash.
- *Meat:* Poultry, fish, shrimp.
- *Fruit:* Orange, banana, grapes, strawberries, raspberries, blackberries, cherries.
- *Foods to Avoid:* Meat or fish for breakfast, spicy and sour foods, deep-fried meat or poultry with a high content of cholesterol and glucose.

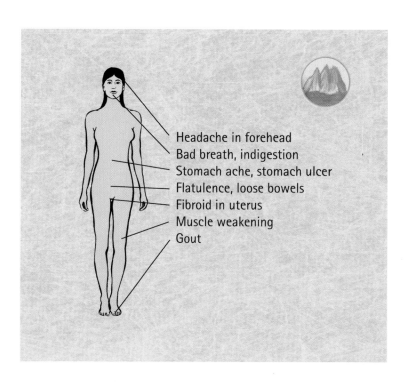

Headache in forehead
Bad breath, indigestion
Stomach ache, stomach ulcer
Flatulence, loose bowels
Fibroid in uterus
Muscle weakening
Gout

Healing Foods for Metal People

Health Disorders or Chronic Complaints Related to the Element of "Metal"

Coughing, asthma, reduced immune reaction, frequent flu, respiratory problems, swelling chest, allergies, stuffy nose, dry skin, thinning of the hair, sore throat, excessive smoking.

Foods with Healing Properties for "Metal":

- *Grain:* Corn, sorghum
- *Legume:* Soybean
- *Vegetable:* Turnip, winter melon, ginger, mushroom, cucumber, string bean, spinach, white cabbage
- *Meat:* Lamb, chicken, rabbit, duck
- *Fruit:* Pineapple, pear, banana, apple, lemon, orange, grapefruit
- *Foods to Avoid:* Chili peppers, pepper, squid, crab

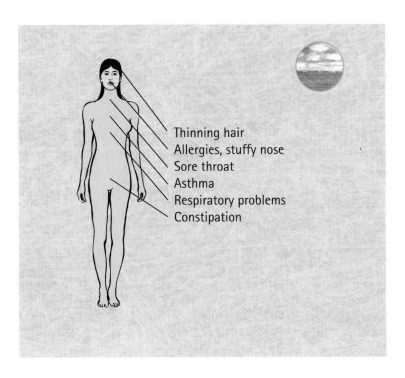

Thinning hair
Allergies, stuffy nose
Sore throat
Asthma
Respiratory problems
Constipation

Healing Foods for Water People

Health Disorders or Chronic Complaints Related to the Element of "Water"

Lumbar pain, protrusion of lumbar vertebral disc, irregular menstrual cycle, polyuria, bladder inflammation, chronic nephritis, male sexual dysfunction, impotence, premature ejaculation, tinnitus, periodontitis.

Foods with Healing Properties for "Water":

- *Grain:* Coarse rice, spaghetti, linseed
- *Legumes:* Beans sprouts, tofu
- *Vegetable:* White cabbage, yam, potato, cauliflower, mushroom, black sesame
- *Meat:* Beef, chicken, lamb, mussels
- *Fruit:* Peaches, grapes, grapefruit, cantaloupe, honeydew, blueberries, strawberries
- *Foods to Avoid:* Monosodium glutamate, salty fish, marinated or smoked foods, alcoholic beverages, chili peppers

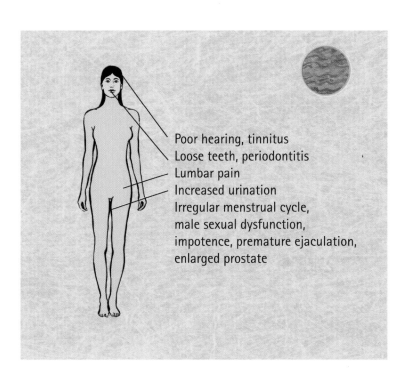

Poor hearing, tinnitus
Loose teeth, periodontitis
Lumbar pain
Increased urination
Irregular menstrual cycle,
male sexual dysfunction,
impotence, premature ejaculation,
enlarged prostate

Healing Foods for Wood People

Health Disorders or Chronic Complaints Related to the Element of "Wood"

Frequent nightmares, insomnia, bad breath, dry mouth and bitter taste in mouth, hypomania, easily stressed, dry eyes, itchy skin, hemorrhoids, arthritis, dizziness, freckles, pimple, pale face, constipation, poor ability to excrete toxins, fatigue, deteriorated eyesight.

Foods with Healing Properties for "Wood"

- *Legume:* Tofu
- *Vegetables:* Spinach, tomato, pumpkin, white cabbage, cauliflower, cucumber, onion
- *Meat:* Duck, liver, fish, other seafood
- *Fruit:* Watermelon, apple, peaches
- *Foods to avoid:* Meat with high cholesterol and acidity, alcoholic beverages, cigarettes, egg yolks

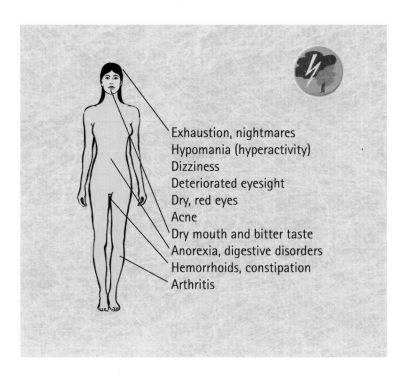

Exhaustion, nightmares
Hypomania (hyperactivity)
Dizziness
Deteriorated eyesight
Dry, red eyes
Acne
Dry mouth and bitter taste
Anorexia, digestive disorders
Hemorrhoids, constipation
Arthritis

Diagnosing Illness through the Hands and Fingers

The hand is like a mirror that reflects the condition of our health: The unhealthy parts of the body are depicted in the palm of the hands and the fingers. Because the ten fingers are connected with the end points of the qi/blood circulation and distribution of meridian routes, any existing problems will be reflected in the fingers as well.

If, for example, a woman has a curve on her little finger, experience has shown that this is related to her reproductive system. This may include an abnormal menstrual cycle and possible gynecological problems.

All health problems are also reflected in the fingers

Both hands act as a magnetic field in our body. The polarities between the backs of the hands (three yang meridians) and the palms of the hands (three yin meridians), together with the starting points of six meridians are prime factors that can affect our health.

We frequently read the signs in the hands to both diagnose disease and treat it with methods of hand healing. Although this method is quite simple, it is also convenient and effective. Daily hand massages, together with healing through specific hand signs and finger movements, contribute to stimulating the hands. In turn, this activates positive functions throughout the entire body.

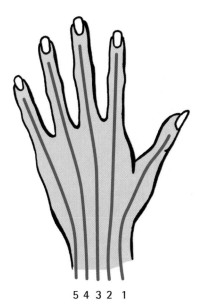

5 4 3 2 1

The energy meridians of the hands
1. *Thumb line*
2. *Index finger line*
3. *Middle finger line*
4. *Ring finger line*
5. *Little finger line*

1. *Strengthening of lungs, elimination of toxic energy*
2. *Regulation of liver, stomach, pancreas, and large intestine*
3. *Regulation of heart and circulatory system*
4. *Regulation of nervous system, vision, sense of equilibrium, stimulation of hormones*
5. *Strengthening*

- **Thumb**

  Hand Tai-Yin of the lung meridian: has supportive effect on respiratory system; enhances the rate of metabolism; helps relieve coughing, asthma, dry mouth, tightness in chest, shoulder and back pain.

- **Index finger**

  Hand Yang-Ming of large intestine meridian: has supportive effect on the liver, stomach, and large intestine; relieves loose bowels, stuffy nose, and laryngitis.

- **Middle finger**

  Hand Jai-Yin of exterior heart meridian: has supportive effect on regulation of blood vessels and circulatory system; helps control tachycardia, irregular heart palpitation, mental disturbances, and problems relaxed to thorax membrane.

- **Ring finger**

  Hand Shao-Yang of triple heater meridian: has supportive effect on tuning of central nervous system, including eye and ear disorders and facial swelling.

- **Little finger**

  Hand Shao-Yin of heart meridian, hand Shao-Yang of small intestine meridian: has supportive effect on regulation of the urinary and reproductive system, including white spots in the eyes; helps relieve shoulder and lumbar pain.

Diagnosing disease through the hands

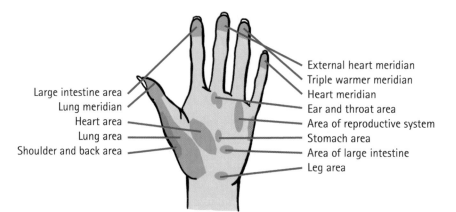

Large intestine area
Lung meridian
Heart area
Lung area
Shoulder and back area

External heart meridian
Triple warmer meridian
Heart meridian
Ear and throat area
Area of reproductive system
Stomach area
Area of large intestine
Leg area

Healing with the Qi Code of the Mudras

According to the theory of meridians in TCM, the ten fingers are connected with the heart. Of the twelve meridian channels in the body, six are located in the hands and fingertips: the three yang and three yin meridians. By holding the hands and bending the fingers in a certain manner, you can regulate the qi and its flow within these meridian channels.

We have adopted an ancient esoteric technique for using special hand signs—also called *mudras*—to regulate and treat body/mind disorders. This method has proved to be both simple and effective. Mudras are a series of established hand positions that support our mind in entering into a tranquil state. They are effective by increasing the unification of body and mind. In the Buddhist wall paintings of the Chinese silk road (*Deun Hwang*), we have discovered many different mudras that are used with meditation. The following five illustrations have been chosen because they show graceful, artistic, and poetic forms of mudras, as well as representing the attunement of each part of the body.

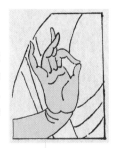

- Qi code of the mudra for "fire" people (sitting position):
  Face north. Men should hold the left hand, women should hold the right hand as shown in the illustration. The other hand rests on the front of the body at the center of the thorax (between the neck and the diaphragm). Inhale deeply through the nose and exhale flatly out of the mouth. Meditate in this position for 20 minutes.

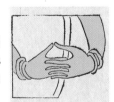

- Qi code of the mudra for "earth" people (prone position):
  Imitate the hand position in the adjacent drawing. Both thumbs should point toward the east just below the navel. Interlace the remaining fingers and place them on your belly. Inhale flatly through the nose and exhale in long breaths. Practice this position for 15 minutes.

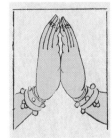

- Qi code of the mudra for "metal" people (sitting position):
  Select an area in quiet surroundings with fresh air and face west. Turn both hands toward each other, leaving the palms hollow. Hold both hands in front of your belly. Inhale simultaneously through your nose and your mouth. Meditate for 10 minutes in this position.

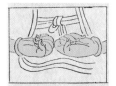

- **Qi code of the mudra for "water" people (sitting position):**
  Face south. Clasp both hands like a fist with the back of the hands facing downward. Rest the hands on top of the thigh. Inhale through your nose, exhale through your mouth. Meditate for 20 minutes in this position.

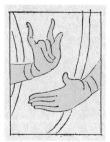

- **Qi code of the mudra for "wood" people (sitting position):**
  Look toward the east. Imitate the hand position in the adjacent illustration. Place the left hand below the rib cage and the right hand in front of the stomach. Inhale flatly through the nose and exhale deeply through your mouth. Meditate for 10 minutes in this position.

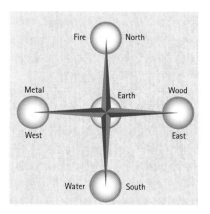

Orientation during exercises and meditation:

Fire people: *North*
Wood people: *East*
Water people: *South*
Metal people: *West*
Earth people: *Toward the sky*

Here are some special hand-massage points for weight control and against back pain and lumbar pain, constipation, insomnia, as well as prevention of the flu. By massaging the shaded points on the following illustrations, you can do your own treatments at home.

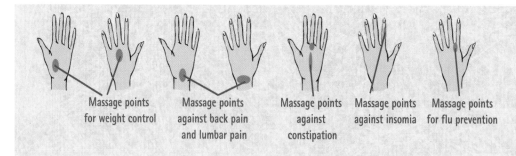

Massage points for weight control | Massage points against back pain and lumbar pain | Massage points against constipation | Massage points against insomia | Massage points for flu prevention

Qi Code for Good Fortune and Spiritual Well-Being

We have found a general tendency while teaching qigong to thousands of students through the years. Particularly the first time that they come to class, they show a variety of expressions on their faces: some are open-minded, some are anxious, and others are suspicious. They are frequently afflicted with pain and health disorders. Some have problems with their family or their work. In general, they bring some type of burden with them. However, after the class is over, the negative and harmful qi in their bodies has been transformed into positive and healing qi.

Negative and toxic qi is eliminated from the body through qigong

Even after the first hour of class, many of the previous conditions change dramatically. Their moods and spiritual/emotional lives are attuned to a clearer and lighter frame of mind. Like lights on a stage that range from dark shadows to full brightness, the previous state of low energy can be transformed into vitality, the previous dullness into agility and lively motion.

Negative moods actually generate negative signals in the mind. With such a pessimistic mental state, we do not enjoy the beautiful plants and flowers or the sounds of nature and the song of the birds. By changing this negative mood into a positive state of mind, we see our immediate surroundings and external circumstances in a more optimistic manner. This leads to the enjoyment of a new, more lively and brighter environment.

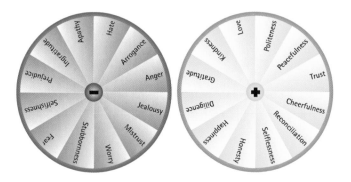

Negative mental signs: disease, poverty, chaos, and misfortune

Positive mental signs: health, peace, stability, and good fortune

The Qi Codes for Success in Business and Prosperity

A lack of qi leads to poor concentration

When we have insufficient qi in our life, this accelerates the aging process. It leads to a lack of mental concentration, dismal feelings about the future, and a feeling of despair. In contrast, when we are filled with positive qi we are pleasant, lively, vibrant, and open-minded. Moreover, we live in harmony with ourselves, create good fortune for ourselves, and also influence others in this direction.

Once the qi in the body has been properly attuned, it actually behaves as if its pattern and flow has been changed. As a result, the telepathic signals in our mind are different as well.

In business life, we should never give up when difficult circumstances arise because qi constantly alters its flow: it can change from good to bad and vice versa. When we do qigong, we particularly focus on the change of bodily qi from weak to strong, from too little to abundant. This transforms the general condition of the body and personality. It can also change our luck, bring good fortune, and enhance the overall quality of our physical lives.

Success occurs when our qi can flow freely

We have adapted to the model of nature and the normal flowing state of qi. When we observe these rules, we can attain a positive change of the qi and ultimately improve our higher thought functions. When we achieve this, our entire life can take on a more optimistic perspective. The moment that we treat other people and the things that surround us with love and a grateful heart, our own qi becomes attuned to the nature of qi. This creates a calm and peaceful atmosphere around us.

In summary, we can say that when nature takes its course, the qi in our bodies will follow its own proper course. This will change every aspect of our lives in a positive way. It is the secret of bringing good fortune, success in business, and prosperity into our lives.

CHAPTER 4

The Five-Elements Rejuvenation Exercises According to Gao Yun

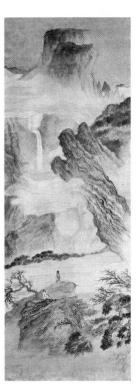

Characteristic Qualities of the Five-Element Rejuvenation Exercises

In general, deviating bodily functions can be attuned through self-adjustment and restored to their normal state of functioning. However, when the organism becomes weak and is incapable of performing this process of self-adjustment, it is necessary to provide external treatment by way of the five elements. A combination of qigong, geomancy (feng shui), nutritional healing, magnetic healing, and mental healing can be effectively used to regulate and balance the bodily dysfunction.

The following exercises are based on the theory of the five elements. They have been compiled in relation to the pathology and physiology of the human body for the purpose of healing with qigong. For healthy individuals, this practice enables the continuous flow of the five elements and a holistic equilibrium of the body. For people who are not completely healthy, this practice will qualitatively enhance the state of the body/mind and prevent disease. For those who are ill, the practice will help them ease the affliction of disease and restore the health of the body/mind.

Five-element qigong according to Gao Yun is a unique exercise that imitates the gestures and movements of five long-living animals. It mainly has the purpose of restoring the balance of yin and yang to the entire body. When practicing the five-element qigong, pay attention to the following three types of regulation:

- **Regulation of posture:** In order to capture the essence of the animal's posture, each movement represents a separate character trait of a long-living animal. Examples of this are the strength of the tiger, the swiftness of the monkey, the joyous flight of the flamingo, the firmness of the bear, and the peacefulness of the deer.
- **Regulation of the mind (visualization):** When practicing the movements, visualize the expression of the animal and become one with it. For example, as you practice the flight of the flamingo, also visualize how you are flying through the air with a joyful, free, and peaceful spirit.

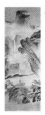

• **Regulation of Vitality:** We imitate not only the posture, but also each animal's unique form of expression. For example, when we practice the Tiger Exercise, we focus on the tiger's claws and imitate them together with the awe-inspiring expression in its eyes and its powerful vitality.

The Characteristics of the Five-Element Exercises

火

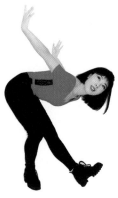

Five-element exercise:	**Fire Exercise**
Organ to be strengthened:	Heart
Animal to imitate:	Flamingo
Animal gestures:	Suppleness, lightness, like wings in flight
Vital expression:	Lightness, suppleness, joyful and serene spirit
Type of visualization:	Joyful, pleasant feeling
Reaction of the body:	Warming of the entire body, sweating— especially on the head
Reaction of the five head openings:	Trembling of the tongue, sounds from the mouth

土

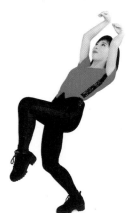

Five-element exercise:	**Earth Exercise**
Organ to be strengthened:	Spleen
Animal to imitate:	Monkey
Animal gestures:	Curling of the limbs, titillation, head tucked in, wiggling the shoulders
Vital expression:	Agility of monkey, active, nimble, and versatile
Type of visualization:	Versatility and swiftness
Reaction of the body:	Warm sensation in the chest and abdomen
Reaction of the five head openings:	Mouth movements, belching

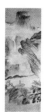

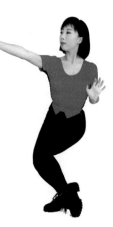

Five-element exercise:	**Metal Exercise**
Organ to be strengthened:	Lungs
Animal to imitate:	Tiger
Animal gestures:	Power and swiftness of the tiger while hunting its prey
Vital expression:	Large tiger eyes, wide-open mouth
Type of visualization:	Majestic dignity and courage
Reaction of the body:	Face and chest feel light and relaxed
Reaction of the five head openings:	Reactions of nose and larynx, flow of phlegm and mucous

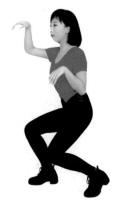

Five-element exercise:	**Water Exercise**
Organ to be strengthened:	Kidneys
Animal to imitate:	Bear
Animal gestures:	Stoutness and firmness of bear, strong upper body, bent at waist
Vital expression:	Drooping eyelids, relaxed face
Type of visualization:	Great refinement and elasticity
Reaction of the body:	Sweating on the back, warm feeling in lower back area
Reaction of the five head openings:	Movement of nose, swelling eardrum

木

Five-element exercise:	**Wood Exercise**
Organ to be strengthened:	Liver
Animal to imitate:	Deer
Animal gestures:	Leaping deer, wiggling head, swinging tail
Type of visualization:	Calm and peaceful
Reaction of the body:	Relaxed mood, feeling of suppleness, slight numbness in limbs, sensation of warmth
Reaction of the five body openings:	Reactions of the eyes, running tears

The circle of the five elements and their associations

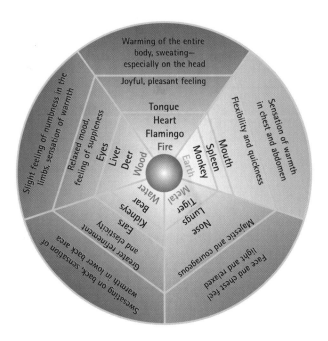

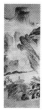

Conspicuous Reactions While Practicing Five-Elements Rejuvenation Exercises

The five-elements rejuvenation exercises lead to quick and powerful results:

1. Certain parts of the body will experience warmth, numbness, and swelling sensations; the temperature will increase in various locations.

2. The organs of the face (eyes, ears, nose, mouth, and tongue) serve as a window leading to the respective vital organs. While practicing the exercise, the vital organs receive the positive results, which are also expressed in the related facial organ.

   Reactions of the improved flow of qi

3. These are positive signs that the stimulating and strengthening energy is received through the practice of the five-element rejuvenation exercise. "Wherever the qi travels, it removes the blocks."

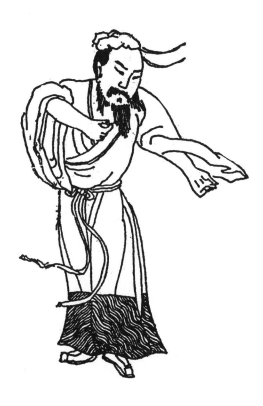

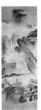

Special Mudras for the Five-Element Rejuvenation Exercises

Each of the five-element rejuvenation exercises according to Gao Yun is designed for a specific purpose. The difference between the hand signs and forms of the mudras is explained by the activation of the relevant meridian channel for the regulation of the qi and the healing of disease. These mudras are specifically intended for the practice of the five-elements rejuvenation exercises.

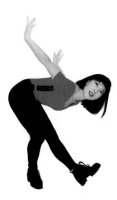
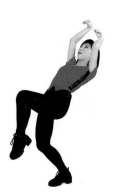

Five-Element Exercise:	Fire Exercise	Earth Exercise
Animal:	Flamingo	Monkey
Mudra:	Flamingo wings	Money hand
Main Theme of Mudra:	Middle finger points downward, connecting with thumb to make a circle; other fingers point upward; small finger points as far up as possible	Make a fist with a hollow palm; round back of hand; tip of thumb lightly touches top part of index finger
Purpose:	Stimulation of the heart and pericardial meridian, strengthening of vessels	Attracting, absorbing, and replenishing qi

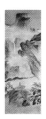

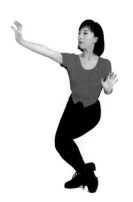 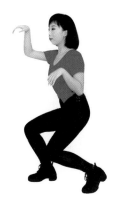 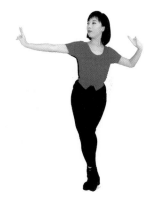

Metal Exercise	Water Exercise	Wood Exercise
Tiger	Bear	Deer
Tiger claw	Bear shape	Deer feet
Bend five fingers into grasping form; slight pressure on thumb and index finger	Make a fist with a hollow palm; round back of hand; tip of thumb lightly touches bottom part of index finger	Middle and index fingers are extended, remaining fingers are bent inward; thumbs are close to index and little fingers
Stimulation of lung and large intestine meridian for elimination of toxic qi	Toning of kidneys, strengthening of waist area, charging of sexual energy, weight control	Cleansing of the liver and gallbladder meridian; facilitates flow of liver qi; relieves pressure; improves sleep

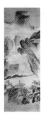
Preparatory Steps for the Five-Elements Rejuvenation Exercises

Before you start the exercises, assume the standing position for Gao Yun Qigong. The purpose of this position is to achieve a balance of yin and yang and allow the qi and the blood to flow freely. This position also supports mental concentration and inner tranquility.

Pay attention to the following details for this position:
- *Feet:* Both feet stand parallel to each other at shoulder width; tilt the body slightly forward
- *Legs:* Bend knees slightly forward
- *Trunk:* Keep chest hollow, tuck in lower abdomen, and relax waist area
- *Shoulders:* Let both shoulders hang down naturally, slightly loosen armpits
- *Head:* Hold head straight and still, eyes face straight ahead
- *Mouth:* Relax mouth, breathe normally

Standing position in Gao-Yun Qigong

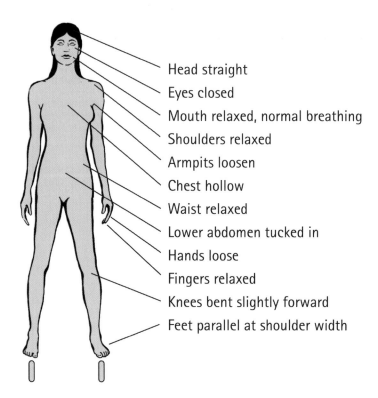

Head straight
Eyes closed
Mouth relaxed, normal breathing
Shoulders relaxed
Armpits loosen
Chest hollow
Waist relaxed
Lower abdomen tucked in
Hands loose
Fingers relaxed
Knees bent slightly forward
Feet parallel at shoulder width

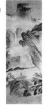

1—The Flamingo Exercise: Qigong for the Fire Element

The Purpose of the Flamingo Exercise

The heart meridian, which is connected with the heart, is the source of vitality for the body and the ultimate protection for life. The heart meridian governs our central nervous system and circulatory system. The Flamingo Exercise helps harmonize the heart meridian; it strengthens the functioning of the heart, relieves stress, helps clear the mind, and balances the qi.

Healing Effects for the Following Symptoms

Neurasthenia, insomnia, dizziness, arrhythmia, arteriosclerosis, palpitation, shortness of breath, weakness, rheumatoid heart disease, hypertension, myocardial oxygen shortness, excessive phlegm, soreness of arms, shoulders and back, nightmare, short memory, dry mouth, still tongue.

Symptoms related to the heart meridian are relieved

Main Reactions to the Flamingo Exercise

- General warming of the body, slight sweating: These are signs that the blood and qi are circulating freely in the body.
- Pleasant and euphoric feelings; the body is filled with vitality and vibrancy; the ultimate goal is harmoniously attuning the heart meridian.

The Names of the Exercises

- Spreading the Wings
- Drinking Water
- Completion Exercise

The Individual Steps of Each Movement

1. Spreading the Wings

- Breathe normally and evenly with a peaceful mind. Visualize how both of your arms are turning into the wings of a flamingo as they move gently and lightly through the air.
- Slightly bend your left leg and point the tip of the left foot downward. Cross your wrists and, with the right hand on top, place them in front of your abdomen.
- Slowly raise your left leg, keeping the knee bent. Move your left thigh toward your chest as you keep the calf and toes pointing downward.
- Form your hands into the shape of flamingo claws to activate the heart meridian. Spread your shoulders like flamingo wings on both sides of your body. While raising both arms into the air, visualize yourself flying upward with your feathers flapping. Simultaneously stretch your head, neck, and spine while keeping your chest and head upright.
- Slowly lower your arms and left leg. Return your hands to the crossed position in front of the abdomen (right hand above, left hand below) and do the above sequence three times. Then switch to the right leg and again do the sequence three times on that side. While ascending, focus on stretching your entire body as much as possible. Then relax as you focus on descending. This will create a balance of yin and yang within you.

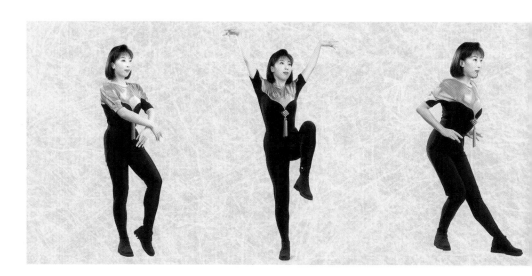

2. Drinking Water

- After you have completed the three sequences with the right leg, take one step forward with the left leg. Lean back and squat down. Shift your body weight to the right leg, bend it slightly, and keep the left leg stretched out in front of you. Assume a sitting posture while keeping the upper body straight. Hold both hands close at waist height with the palms facing downward.

- Lean your body forward, turn the palms upward with all ten fingers pointing behind you. Then raise both arms from the back of the body and keep them extended.

- Now make flattering motions with your hands, keeping the palms facing upward. As you do this, slowly let your hands descend from the back of the waist to your feet as if you were drawing a semicircle of 180 degrees. Then slowly raise the front of your body. When both hands are at chest height, shift the weight of your body onto the front position of the left leg. Now bend the front leg and stretch the back leg.

- Slowly bring both hands to your waist. Stretch your chest and raise your head. When you shift your body weight back to your right leg, one sequence of Drinking Water has been completed.

- Now move the right leg one step forward and shift your body weight to your other leg. Do the entire exercise sequence three times.

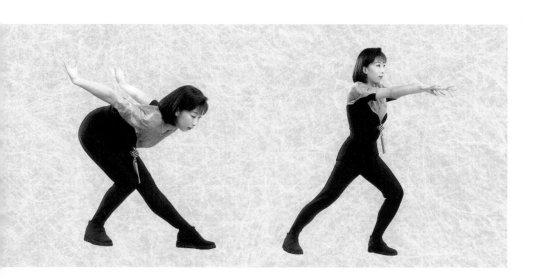

3. Completion Exercise

Move the left leg one step forward and return to the initial standing position of the Flamingo Exercise.

Pay Special Attention to these Aspects of the Flamingo Exercise

- Continue to do the flattering hand movement of the flamingo wing from the first step of the exercise to the concluding movement.
- During the "wing-spreading" part of the exercise, focus your attention on visualizing how your arms have bird's feathers on them. Experience how light you are as you soar through the air.
- Breathe in a normal and stable rhythm, but not too quickly. Coordinate your movements with your breathing: Inhale while ascending and exhale while descending.

The Secrets of a Healthy Lifestyle for Fire People

Strengthening of the heart meridian and relief from heart complaints through the Flamingo Exercise

Disorders of the heart meridian are normally associated with fire people. Symptoms usually occur around noon in the form of slight nervous heart trouble, respiratory difficulties, or a weak form of tinnitus. People who have heart problems should avoid physical exercise, including the Flamingo Exercise, during the midday hours. It is best to remain calm during this time, which will support a reduction of excessive heat in the heart.

Since the heart is associated with the "fire" of the five elements, its respective position is north. Consequently, people with problems of the heart or circulatory system will fear winter and cold nights. This is expressed in mild symptoms such as chilly hands and feet; the most severe form is myocardial infarction, which usually occurs during the coldest nights. Practicing the Flamingo Exercise during the winter can prevent a worsening of heart problems and maintain the proper flow of energy in the heart meridian. This promotes a healthy lifestyle.

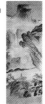

2—The Monkey Exercise: Qigong for the Earth Element

The Purpose of the Monkey Exercise

The Monkey Exercise mainly regulates the stomach and spleen meridian. This influences the intake of nutrients and their transformation into important bodily substances such as blood, lymph, and saliva. The stomach and spleen are primary energy sources for the body. They are the most important digestive organs and responsible for absorbing and conveying nutrients throughout the body. When the functions of the stomach and spleen are disturbed, the body's energy level will begin to deteriorate. This occurrence is expressed in a pale face and can lead to physical complaints. Proper functioning of the stomach and spleen support and intensify the body's life essence, which is displayed in an improved condition of the skin and prevention of strokes.

Healing Effects for the Following Symptoms

Excessive flatulence, gastritis, stomach ulcer, gastroptosis, duodenal ulcer, anorexia, ascites, vomiting, stomach ache, fatigue, poor digestion, functional disturbances of stomach and spleen, constipation, chronic hepatitis, stroke, diabetes, cancer of the colon, rheumatic arthritis, gallstone, eating disorders that may include hunger, inadequate eating that leads to insufficient qi and blood, which reduces the immune response and makes the body more susceptible to diseases.

Relief of symptoms related to the stomach and spleen

Main Reactions to the Monkey Exercise

- A numb and itchy feeling in the body is the result of qi/blood reaching the surface skin area
- Increased saliva, more bowel activity, better appetite, and a sweeter taste when eating are signs of a stimulated metabolism
- Warm, prickling sensation around the mouth and perineum area is the result of the body detoxifying negative energy.

Names of the exercises:
- *Rubbing the Ears*
- *Circling the Qi Ball*
- *Completion Exercise*

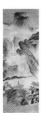

The Individual Steps of Each Movement

1. Rubbing the Ears

- Breathe slowly and evenly. Visualize the characteristics of a monkey such as activity, swiftness, scratching movements, and a state of constant agility.
- Shift your body weight to your left foot. Arch the right foot to activate the stomach meridian. Form a monkey hand with your fingers and place your hands on both sides of your lower abdomen. The palms should face upward and the fingers pointing at each other.
- From the front of the body, raise the right hand and brush it along the left side of the chest until it reaches the left earlobe and moves behind it. Tilt the body forward with the chest hollow and the stomach tucked in. Contract the neck.
- Move the right hand past the back of the head. As you do this, let the little finger trace down the right side of the chest to the waist while the other fingers point upward.
- After you have done this movement three times, change sides and let the left hand stroke over the right ear three times. Then let both hands, with palms facing upward, rest on your lower abdomen.

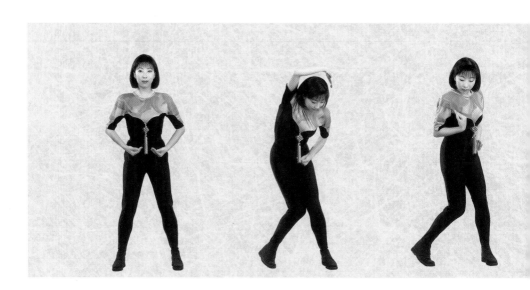

2. Circling the Qi Ball

- Slowly raise both arms away from the body and bring the hands into a position with the right hand above and the left hand below. Both palms face each other as if you were holding a ball of qi in front of your abdomen.
- Turn your body to the left and shift your body weight to the left leg. Slightly bend right leg with the sole touching the ground and the toes of the right foot pointing to the left.
- The left hand is still. Place the right hand above it and do a total of seven circles from the inside to the outside in a *counterclockwise* direction. While forming the circles, let your waist follow the motion. Your body will also turn from left to right while your hands circle it.
- When you have completed the turns to the right, shift your body weight to your right leg. Slightly bend the left leg. Reverse the position of your hands so that the left hand is now above and the right hand is below. Both palms are facing each other, as if you were holding a ball of qi.
- Now do the Circling the Qi Ball Exercise in the other direction, meaning *clockwise*, seven times.
- Then bring your body back to the starting position and hold your hands on your abdomen.

3. Completion Exercise

Let your hands slowly descend and return to the initial standing position.

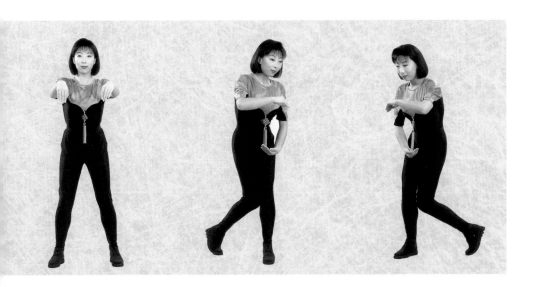

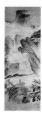

Pay Special Attention to These Aspects of the Monkey Exercise

- It is important to concentrate on the activity and agility, as well as the similarity with the curling and stretching characteristics of the monkey. When you lean forward, let your chest be hollow and contract your abdomen.
- Maintain the form of the monkey hand from the beginning of the exercise to the last movement before returning to the initial standing position.
- When rubbing your ear, feel the earlobe as you pass your face. When you move past the neck and stroke down the chest, concentrate on your fingers pointing upward while the outer part of the little finger touches the body. The overall sensation resembles the scratching of a monkey.
- When you circle the ball, focus on your waist turning and the rest of the body following this motion. Keep your body in a forward position so that the abdomen is massaged by the motion.
- After the exercise, you may experience a gentle, numbing, tickling, prickling, warm, and soothing sensation.

The Secrets of the Healthy Lifestyle for Earth People

One more bit of advice regarding the diet, which is also our favorite motto: a nourishing and protein-rich breakfast, a plentiful and varied lunch, and a very modest dinner (small portion)

Proper care of the stomach and spleen is an important part of a healthy lifestyle. The peak functioning period for the stomach and spleen is between 7 a.m. and 9 a.m., before breakfast. We therefore suggest that you relax during this time and maintain a peaceful mind. Individuals who have problems with the stomach meridian should select very nutritious foods for breakfast such as a variety of grains, but you should avoid meat products. This will provide your body with the necessary energy for its daily consumption.

When you practice this exercise, be sure you do not overeat. Moreover, do not practice immediately after meals. Don't lose your temper while you eat and thoroughly chew your food before swallowing it.

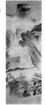

3—Tiger Exercise:
Qigong for the Metal Element

The Purpose of the Tiger Exercise

The lung is the governor of the body. It supports the functioning of the heart (which we could call the president) as it purifies and regulates our organism. The Tiger Exercise mainly strengthens the lung meridian, invigorates the respiratory system, and speeds up the elimination of negative energy from the metabolic process. The lung meridian also regulates the opening and closing of the skin and pores, which helps beautify and tone the skin.

Healing Effects for the Following Symptoms

Susceptibility to flu, weak immune ability, heavy breathing during movement, dull and hoarse voice, sore and swollen throat, inability to hold a prolonged conversation, low and deep sound of the voice in women, high and weak sound of the voice in men, bronchitis, bronchial enlargement, nasal allergy, stuffy nose, excessive phlegm, gasping, frequent sneezing, runny nose, dry skin and hair, excessive wrinkles, frequent hemorrhoids, and difficulty breathing.

Relief of symptoms related to the lung meridian

Main Reactions to the Tiger Exercise

Because the lungs are connected with the skin and pores, the pores will be slightly open after the practice of this exercise. The roots of the hair experience a tickling sensation. For some people, the qi travels through the skin's surface, producing redness and strong skin coloring. For others, this generates moisture in the skin, which can be either cool or warm, including moist nostrils and the discharge of mucous. All of these reactions are part of the body's self-regulation and clearing of the blocked qi.

The names of the exercises:
- *Tiger Claw*
- *Release of Qi*
- *Completion Exercise*

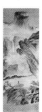

The Individual Steps of Each Movement

1. Tiger Claw

- Assume the initial standing position, breathe normally and evenly, and visualize the tiger's characteristics: full of vitality, power, and majesty.
- Place your hands at both sides of your waist. Rotate your hands and wrists inward seven times to activate the lung meridian.
- Move your left leg forward with one big step. Bend the left leg in the front and keep the right leg in the back straight. Form each hand into a tiger claw and hold at chest height in front of the body. Begin forcefully pushing out the left hand while opening your mouth and making the "ha" sound.
- Slowly bring your left hand back toward your chest. Then push your right hand forward, open your mouth, and make the "ha" sound again. Repeat this sequence with alternate hands seven times in a row (L, R, L, R, L, R, L).
- Move the left leg back and take a big step forward with your right leg. Repeat the above movement by placing your body weight on the front, bend the leg. Form each hand into a tiger claw and hold at chest height in front of the body. Raise your right hand and extend it in front of you. After you have grasped the qi, bring your hand back to your chest. Repeat this sequence with alternate hands seven times in a row (R, L, R, L, R, L, R).

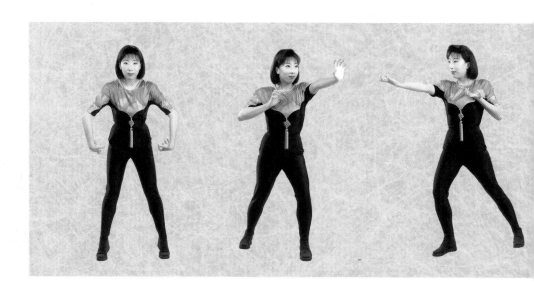

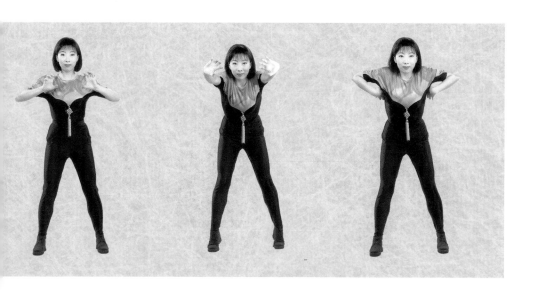

2. Releasing the Qi

- Move the left leg back, but keep the initial form of the standing position.
- Place both hands quietly in front of your chest with the palms of the tiger claws facing forward. Lift the heels of both feet from the floor. As you do this, your weight will shift to the front half of the soles. Bend your body slightly forward.
- Powerfully push both hands forward as you drop your heels to the ground and make the "ha" sound.
- With the backs of your hands facing each other, circle them in an outward direction (like a crawl stroke in swimming). When the hands reach the body, brush through the armpit area and return to the front of the chest.
- Repeat this exercise sequence seven times. Each time you push your hands forward and drop your heals, make the "ha" sound.

3. Completion Exercise

Slowly lower both hands and return to the initial standing position.

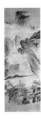

Pay Special Attention to the Following Aspects of the Tiger Exercise

- Hold your hands in the form of tiger claws for the entire exercise.
- Push out the qi with rapid speed and a powerful stroke. This is intended to intensify the discharge of toxic qi from your lungs. When you grasp the qi during the return motion, visualize capturing and pulling the qi back into your lungs.
- The Tiger stance should be firm and solid as a rock. Place your body weight on the front, bent leg while you keep the back leg straight.
- The entire exercise should be done in a stance of powerful strength and majestic dignity. Push the hands out as quick as lightning and then move them back slowly so that the balance of yin and yang is maintained.

The Secrets of a Healthy Lifestyle for Metal People

It has been scientifically proved that the human body tends to have lower blood pressure in the early morning hours between 3 a.m. and 5 a.m. The rate of the pulse and breathing are also reduced during this period. Because of the diminished supply of blood, seizures occur more frequently during this period. Coronary thrombosis and cerebral embolism during this time of day are more likely to lead to sudden death.

On the other hand, the active period for the flow of the qi in the lung meridian is between 3 a.m. and 5 p.m. If the lung qi is strong and plentiful, it will increase the immune ability for fighting negative qi. Practicing the Tiger Exercise during this time period will greatly improve the lungs' ability to function. It also has a positive effect on establishing a healthy lifestyle.

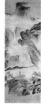

4—The Bear Exercise: Qigong for the Water Element

The Purpose of the Bear Exercise

The main purpose of the Bear Exercise is to regulate the urinary and reproductive system. TCM believes that the kidneys store our bodily essences. The growth and development of the human body, the formation of bone marrow, the reproduction of life—all of these functions depend on the "bio essence" stored in the kidneys.

By strengthening the kidneys, we can increase our lifespan, extend the period of reproductive fertility, enhance sexual functioning, and prolong the "golden age of youth." On the other hand, a weakening of the kidneys leads to various chronic ailments.

Healing Effects for the Following Symptoms

Relief for symptoms related to the kidneys and sexual functions

Disorders of the sexual functions in men and women, impotence, premature ejaculation, irregular menstrual cycle, frigidity, infertility, nephritis, lower back pain, cold feeling in abdomen, weak bladder, polyuria, strangury, cystitis; deterioration of hearing, tinnitus; weakening of both legs, sensation of soreness and pain in entire body, loosening of bones, and aches in bones.

Main Reactions to the Bear Exercise

- Sweating on the back and waist, warm feeling as a result of qi and blood circulation as it reaches the weakest part of the body (back and waist) or the area most likely to be blocked.
- Improved quality of sleep, less dreams as a result of attuning the autonomic nervous system.
- Feeling of tenderness and soreness on the inner part of the thigh due to clearing of the kidney meridian, which leads to the genitals.
- Feeling of moisture in female genitals with a small amount of secretion; warming of the male's penis. Both of these reactions are a result of increased hormone production within the sexual glands.

The names of the exercises
- *Tree Jolt*
- *Treading the Rock*
- *Completion Exercise*

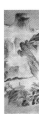
The Individual Steps of the Movement

1. Tree Jolt

- Breathe normally and evenly. First visualize the characteristics of the bear: firmness and solidity, stolid nature, a body that is thick and heavy, powerful and round, with slow and easy motions.
- Bend the upper body forward to waist height. Raise both arms at the same time with the left hand in front at chest height and the right hand in back at waist height. Keep both palms facing the body. Now start swaying back and forth while raising the heel of the right foot and turning the upper body to the right.
- Put the right heel firmly on the ground, lower the left hand, and switch it to the back position. Bring the right hand to the front at chest height while simultaneously raising the heel of the left foot from the ground.
- Do this alternating sequence of letting the arms sway back and forth and the heels lift and drop for a total of seven times.

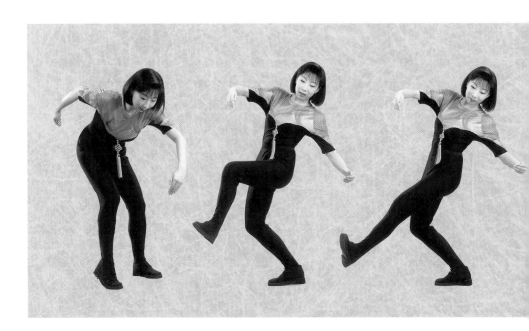

2. Treading the Rock

- The left hand is in front of the body, the right hand behind the body. Both palms are facing the body.
- Raise the left leg and shift the body weight to the right leg, then lean to the left. Both hands hold an invisible circle (ball of qi) on the left side of the body.
- The left foot and toes point upward. With the left heel, perform a hard and firm kick to activate the kidney meridian.
- Lower the left leg to the floor and shift the body weight forward to the left leg. Keep the left leg bent and the right leg straight behind you. Both hands are still in the position of holding the qi ball.
- With the waist leading the upper body, begin swaying to the right and back. Do this exercise sequence three times and then return to the frontward posture.

3. Completion Exercise

During the final phase, let both hands slide downward. Position the feet parallel with each other and return to the initial standing position.

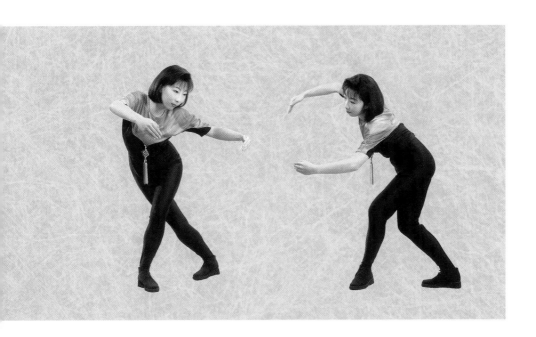

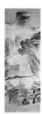

Pay Special Attention to the Following Aspects of the Bear Exercise

- Mainly focus on the movement of the legs. Both legs should remain firm and stable.
- When jolting the tree, imagine how the bear keeps moving in slow motion.
- The swaying of the body should also be done in a slow, strong, and powerful way.
- During the entire exercise, maintain the position of holding the qi ball between the palms as they face each other.
- When doing the Treading the Rock Exercise, maintain firmness and balance. Before you do the kick, tilt your body slightly to the rear. Then kick with the force generated in the heel while treading the rock.

The Secrets of a Healthy Lifestyle for Water People

From the perspective of TCM, the kidneys represent our entire urinary and reproductive system. TCM also believes that the kidneys are the essence of life. We therefore recommend that you protect your kidneys from abuse. The Chinese pay considerable attention to the rules regarding sexual behavior. For example, there are various conditions under which sexual intercourse should be avoided. These include: stormy nights, eclipses of the sun and moon (especially between 1 a.m. and 3 a.m.), excessive alcohol consumption and overeating, serious illness, and during menstruation. Also avoid swimming in contaminated water immediately after intercourse.

Here is a secret for those who frequently suffer from exhaustion and are apathetic toward sexual activities: If a couple wants to have intimate relations, they should massage each other's perineum (area between the anus and genitals). This should be done in a circular motion that is repeated 36 times, which may gradually be increased to 99 times. The fingers should be warmed beforehand. This method enhances the sexual functions during intercourse.

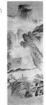

5—The Deer Exercise: Qigong for the Wood Element

The Purpose of the Deer Exercise

The Deer Exercise primarily regulates the liver and the gallbladder. The liver, with its two-fold function of regulating the qi and the blood and eliminating toxic substances within the blood, is one of the crucial organs of the body. In connection with the other vital organs, it also performs the tasks of regulating emotions, reducing stress, and clearing one of the most important channels within the body—the governor meridian, which is the main terminal of all the yang meridians.

Healing Effects for the Following Symptoms

Bad moods, worry and depression, restlessness, deterioration of vision, premature presbyopia, teary eyes, dry eyes; itchy, red iris; disorder of the liver function due to excessive medication, enlargement of the liver, gallstones; back pain, stiff back and shoulders; fatigue.

Relief of the symptoms related to the liver and gallbladder

Main Reactions to the Deer Exercise

- During practice, some people may experience tears. After the practice, our vision is clear and bright as a result of the increased blood circulation to both eyes and detoxification of the qi. The eyes are the windows of the liver meridian. When the liver meridian is blocked, the results may be near-sightedness, cataract, astigmatism, and so forth. A blocked liver meridian also may lead to insomnia, nervousness, hypertension, arthritis, and hemorrhoids.
- Once the liver meridian has been cleared, we can usually experience tranquil emotions, a relaxed body, and a peaceful mind.
- An increased frequency of the bowel movement (but not loose bowels or abdominal pain) is the result of speeding up the processing in which stool deposits are eliminated from the intestines.

The names of the exercises
- *Swinging the Tail*
- *Pointing to the Sky*
- *Completion Exercise*

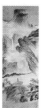
The Individual Steps of Each Movement

1. Swinging the Tail

- Begin with the initial standing position and breathe normally. First visualize the characteristics of the deer: cheerful and friendly, stretching as it leaps and runs, the rocking head and swinging tail.

- Raise both hands together in front of the body at shoulder height and at shoulder width. Let your wrists hang downward and form your fingers into a deer hoof. Then start pointing your fingers upward. Move both hands apart in a horizontal direction until they reach the two sides of the body. Lower them backward and downward, then place your hands on your waist. The index and middle fingers are at the front of the waist, the thumb is at the back of it.

- Using your hips, circle your waist seven times in a counterclockwise direction; then reverse the direction and circle clockwise seven times. While doing this exercise, concentrate the movement on the waist and lower body.

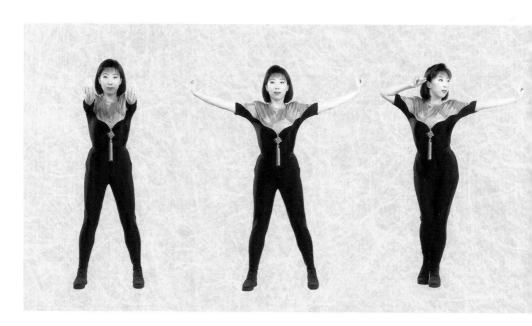

2. Pointing to the Sky

- After completion of the waist circling, once again raise both hands to the sides of the body and extend them. Form the fingers into the shape of a deer hoof and point them upward.
- Let the left foot slightly nudge the inner side of the right foot. The toes should still touch the ground and the body weight is shifted toward the center and downward.
- Bend the left arm toward your left ear, then extend it to the side again. At the same time, bend the right arm toward your right ear. Push the left and right hand outward and back for a total of seven times.
- Change to the right foot. Keep your toes on the ground. Do the entire exercise sequence a total of seven times on this side of the body.

3. Completion Exercise

Lower both hands. Place the feet parallel to each other, and return to the initial standing position.

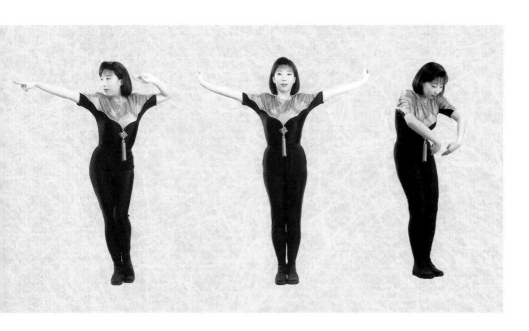

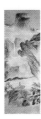

Pay Special Attention to the Following Aspects of the Deer Exercise

- The starting point of the governor meridian is located at the coccyx. While doing the circling hip movement, you should therefore focus on keeping your chest hollow and your abdomen contracted. Bend the knees slightly and point the coccyx downward. A normal reaction to this exercise may be a sore coccyx. Use the coccyx like an axis, around which you circle. Be totally relaxed and do not use any force as you first circle in the counterclockwise direction and then the clockwise direction.
- When stretching out one arm straight at your side, be sure to simultaneously bend the other arm and bring it behind the respective ear. While you push the arm outward, follow the direction and movement of the deer "fingers" with your eyes.
- Maintain a calm mind and balanced mood while you do this exercise.

The Secrets of a Healthy Lifestyle for Wood People

People who frequently suffer from improper sleep or insomnia can drink a glass of warm milk of soak their feet in hot water for 5 to 10 minutes before going to bed. This can support the strengthening of the liver and improve the quality of sleep. The active period for the liver meridian is 1:00 a.m. to 3:00 a.m. Bad habits such as going to bed too late, anxiety, poor nutrition, excessive drinking, and lack of exercise will lead to liver damage. Going to sleep before 11 p.m. will improve the liver meridian's functions and relief the liver from excessive exertion.

Master Gao Yun and Master Bai Yin

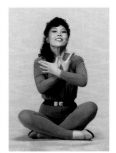

Master Gao Yun is a qigong master of extraordinary radiance, power, and experience. Without a doubt, she is one of the most popular qigong masters in the world. She is a professor at the Peking University, director of the Eastern Qigong Hospital in Peking, chairperson of the International Qigong Institute, and publisher of the *China Qigong Magazine*. From 1985 to the end of the Nineties, she commuted between China and California; today she lives in Taipei and holds training seminars throughout the world. She has introduced more than 300,000 students in 28 countries to qigong.

Her path began many years ago with a Taoist hermit in the remote mountains of China. Today, she is the youngest—and only woman—to be officially recognized by China as a Grand Master of Qigong.

Her *Qi Gong for Life* is a new therapeutic form of qigong: short, simple, but very effective exercises for the healing of hypertension, gastrointestinal complaints, sexual problems, insomnia, overweight, and many more ailments. As a physician, she knows where the greatest problems are; as a qigong master, she has found the most gentle and effective manner of strengthening the life energy, the free flowing of the qi within human beings. This is the best foundation for a comprehensive feeling of well-being, health, and youthful vitality.

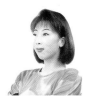

Master Bai Yin has been instructed in qigong since early youth by her mother, Dr. Gao Yun. At the age of 29, she has already made a name for herself as probably the youngest internationally recognized qigong master: she has trained more than 5,000 students to date and holds advanced training courses for qigong in various countries.

At the age of 13, she first came to America with her mother. She later studied at the University of California, from which she graduated with honors. In addition to the many seminars that they lead throughout the world, both mother and daughter work at their center for naturopathy in Taipei, Taiwan.

The qigong seminar series *Qi Gong for Life* includes selected sequences of mental and physical exercises that have a strengthening and invigorating effect on the life energy, qi. This dynamic form of Chinese healing meditation promises agility and youthfulness up to a ripe old age. The exercises are designed to relieve both general and specific health disorders.

The basic course is suitable for participants of all ages, both with and without previous knowledge of qigong. It focuses on highly effective health exercises. *Qi Gong for Life* effectively helps against respiratory and heart problems, diabetes, overweight, gynecological and urological disorders, gastrointestinal complaints, allergies, neck and back pain, colds, and much more. All of the exercises are precisely explained, demonstrated several times, and repeated together. *Qi Gong for Life* offers a great variety of different courses, including advanced and qigong-trainer programs.

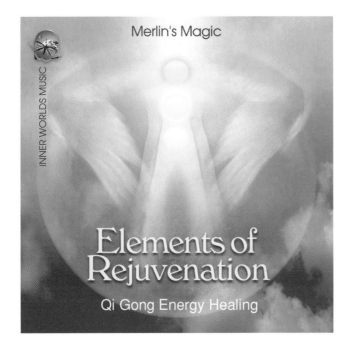

Merlin's Magic

Merlin's Magic
Elements of Rejuvenation

Qi Gong Energy Healing

Qi Gong Energy Healing

This music has been composed especially for Qigong, but it is just as suitable for slow movement exercises such as yoga and t'ai chi. The uplifting melodies flow smoothly in resonance with subtle qi movements and awaken energies that are unexpectedly powerful. Listening to these exceptional qi sounds allows people to become more deeply in touch with the universal life energy, and heal themselves.

Total running length:
60 minutes
CD 41094 • US$17.95
ISBN 0-910261-43-1

The music was composed in synchronization with the performance of the exercises, which concentrate on simple physical movements and can be performed effortlessly. They are also suitable for those who have no previous experience with Qigong.

The meridians will be cleansed, so that the qi can flow freely. The melodies energize the resonance between the inner organs, create synchronous vibrations and cause subtle healing effects.

Coordination with the music is an important element. The movements selected for this album are based on the lectures by Qigong Master Gao Yun and Master Bai Yin.

Smoothly flowing harmonious **melodies** twined with subtle sounds of Far-Eastern instruments.

The album is accompanied by **a booklet**, containing 11 Taoist Qigong exercises and meditation instructions, which can be performed in synchronization with the music.

The following CDs are also suitable for creating and accompanying a relaxing, healing atmosphere:

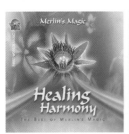

Quiet and pure

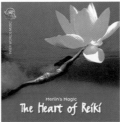

Ideal for Reiki treatment positions

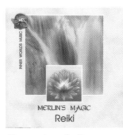

Harmonious feelings

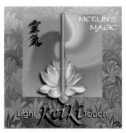

The Reiki classic

Titles Released by LOTUS PRESS · SHANGRI-LA

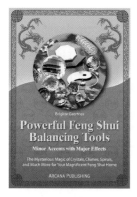

Brigitte Gaertner
Powerful Feng Shui Balancing Tools
Minor Accents with Major Effects
The Mysterious Magic of Crystals, Chimes, Spirals, and Much More for Your Magnificent Feng Shui Home
Powerful Feng Shui Balancing Tools is a standard work, based on the traditional Chinese knowledge, a book that exclusively presents these mysterious accents with powerful effects. A balancing tool consciously placed in the right location of your home exerts concealed positive Chi powers which harmonize the area of its influence, improving the quality of your life, by giving you inner peace, comfort and a long-lasting health.
Minor accents often have major effects and influence your well-being. Balancing tools are thoroughly studied in the feng shui tradition and emerge from old Chinese symbols. Once you have read this book, it will be simple for you to use them for your benefit: put a DNS spiral in your living and working area, hang a dragon picture in a window facing east or place a pair of dolphins in the Relationship Zone... The effects of these graceful tools can accomplish true wonders. Accompanied by a wealth of lovely colored illustrations and pictures, which help you choose the proper accents to energize and clear your home from clutter in such a way, that it becomes a source of flowing Chi.
96 pages · 108 photos · US$14.95
ISBN 0-910261-20-2 · ARCANA PUBLISHING

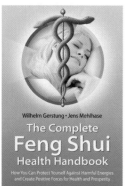

Wilhelm Gerstung · Jens Mehlhase
The Complete Feng Shui Health Handbook
How You Can Protect Yourself against Harmful Energies and Create Positive Forces for Health and Prosperity
The Chinese art of Feng Shui has existed for more than 5,000 years, surrounded by a mysterious and mystical aura. Today, it is a well-known fact that invisible energies have a direct impact on our health and well-being.
This fascinating Feng Shui handbook provides a wealth of graphics and practical information, which help design every home in such a way that it becomes a source of energy, allowing everybody to relax and re-energize himself.
Wilhelm Gerstung and Jens Mehlhase are experienced Feng Shui practitioners and consultants. They explain how the invisible energies of Feng Shui can be directly measured and evaluated using a tensor (single-handed dowser) or pendulum. This means that you can use Feng Shui to understand many health problems by relating them to energy imbalances. The authors integrate their many years of research and extensive knowledge of energies in the home, and particularly the sleeping area, with the Western science of underground watercourses and grids. They have advanced this knowledge in relation to Feng Shui.
224 pages · US$16.95 · ISBN 0-914955-60-8

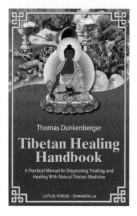

Thomas Dunkenberger
Tibetan Healing Handbook
A Practical Manual for Diagnosing, Treating, and Healing with Natural Tibetan Medicine
An introduction to one of the oldest healing systems: Tibetan natural medicine—comprehensive and easy to understand.
The author informs you about the essential correlations and approaches taken by the Tibetan science of healing. He describes the entire spectrum of application possibilities for those who want to study Tibetan medicine and use it for treatment purposes.
Tibetan Healing Handbook discusses the fundamental principles of health and causes of disease. These include non-visible forces and biorhythmic-planetary influences; classic Tibetan forms of diagnosis, the foremost of which are pulse and urine examination; advice on behavior and healing approaches to dietary habits, as well as the accessory therapeutic possibilities of oil massages, moxabustion, hydrotherapy, humoral excretion procedures, and famous Tibetan remedies.
240 pages · US$15.95 · ISBN 0-914955-66-7

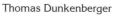

Titles Released by LOTUS PRESS · SHANGRI-LA

Barbara Simonsohn
Barley Grass Juice
Rejuvenation Elixir and Natural, Healthy Power Drink
Easy to Prepare and Totally Healthy, Barley Grass Juice Works True Wonders
A Perfect Food with a Complete Complex of Vital Substances
There's finally a totally healthy "fast food"—as barley grass juice is called by Dr. Yoshihi-de Hagiwara, the Japanese authority on barley grass juice. Prepared quickly, it is an optimal supplement to the daily diet. Barley grass juice has an excellent nutrient profile and many advantages over wheat grass juice. It is a perfect food with a complete complex of vital substances. Barley grass has unimagined healing possibilities that not only confirm everything that we have known up to now about it but also exceed it. Barley grass juice is also a very good preparation and accompanying therapy for the optimal use of any type of homeopathy.
Expert Barbara Simonsohn reveals the secrets of this effective green elixir, including the experiences of barley grass pioneers and a large spectrum of recipes.
160 pages · US$14.95 • ISBN 0-914955-68-3

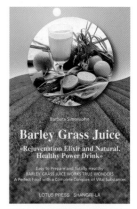

Walter Lübeck · Frank Arjava Petter · William Lee Rand
The Spirit of Reiki
Written by three world-renowned Reiki masters, The Spirit of Reiki is a first. Never before have three Reiki masters from different lineages and with such extensive background come together to write a book and share their experience. *The Spirit of Reiki* contains a wealth of information on Reiki never before brought together in one place. The broad spectrum of topics range from the search for a scientific explanation of Reiki energy to Reiki as a spiritual path. It includes the latest understanding of Dr. Usui's original healing methods, how Reiki is currently practiced in Japan, an analysis of the Western evolution of Reiki, and a discussion about the direction Reiki is likely to take in the future.
A definition of Reiki is included along with class outlines, an in depth analysis of the Reiki symbols and a discussion of the teacher/student relationship. Chapters about Dr. Mikao Usui, Chujiro Hayashi, Hawayo Takata, and other important figures, supplemented by original writings, make this book an important document of contemporary Reiki history. An additional 20 Usui treatment positions, which have not been previously published, along with the Hayahsi Healing Guide complete this book as a compendium of Reiki knowledge.
312 pages · 150 b/w illustrations · US$19.95 • ISBN 0-914955-67-5

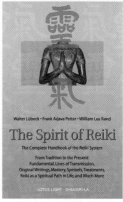

Dr. Mikao Usui and Frank Arjava Petter
The Original Reiki Handbook of Dr. Mikao Usui
For the First Time Available outside Japan: The Traditional Usui Reiki Ryoho Treatment Positions and Numerous Reiki Techniques for Health and Well-Being
Seventy-three years after the death of Reiki's founder, his handbook—a document that he gave to all of his students to accompany them on their path during his lifetime—is now available. With its help, each of us can directly connect with Mikao Usui and his system of Reiki. Many people who practice Reiki will experience this as a spiritual weight off of their minds: Some of the things that we have silently felt, thought, or even practiced on our own are now personally blessed by the founder of Reiki. With simple steps that are easy to understand, Dr. Usui shows us how specific parts of the body and health disorders can be treated successfully. He gives our hands the freedom to move to where they are needed and teaches us to purify our minds through meditation and breathing exercises. Intuition—which has frequently been a neglected tool in Western Reiki up to now—is valued and honored here. This creates a completely "new" picture of Reiki that will considerably deepen our understanding, no matter what degree of Reiki we have learned.
Illustrated with approximately one hundred beautiful color photographs that reflect the spirit of Reiki and accurately depict the respective positions.
80 pages · full color · US$14.95 • ISBN 0-914955-57-8

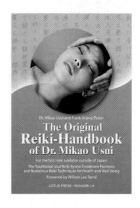

Herbs and other natural health products and information are often available at natural food stores or metaphysical bookstores. If you cannot find what you need locally, you can contact one of the following sources of supply.

Sources of Supply:

The following companies have an extensive selection of useful products and a long track-record of fulfillment. They have natural body care, aromatherapy, flower essences, crystals and tumbled stones, homeopathy, herbal products, vitamins and supplements, videos, books, audio tapes, candles, incense and bulk herbs, teas, massage tools and products and numerous alternative health items across a wide range of categories.

WHOLESALE:

Wholesale suppliers sell to stores and practitioners, not to individual consumers buying for their own personal use. Individual consumers should contact the RETAIL supplier listed below. Wholesale accounts should contact with business name, resale number or practitioner license in order to obtain a wholesale catalog and set up an account.

Lotus Light Enterprises, Inc.

P. O. Box 1008
Silver Lake, WI 53170 USA
262 889 8501 (phone)
262 889 8591 (fax)
800 548 3824 (toll free order line)

RETAIL:

Retail suppliers provide products by mail order direct to consumers for their personal use. Stores or practitioners should contact the wholesale supplier listed above.

Internatural

33719 116th Street
Twin Lakes, WI 53181 USA
800 643 4221 (toll free order line)
262 889 8581 office phone
WEB SITE: www.internatural.com

Web site includes an extensive annotated catalog of more than 10,000 products that can be ordered "on line" for your convenience 24 hours a day, 7 days a week.